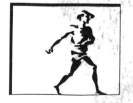

LOOKING GOOD, FEELING BEAUTIFUL

The Avon Book of Beauty

Art Direction & Design by John Staiano
Photographs by Charles Tracy

Simon and Schuster
Avon Products, Inc.
New York

Copyright © 1981 by Avon Products, Inc.
All rights reserved
including the right of reproduction
in whole or in part in any form
Published by Simon and Schuster
A Division of Gulf & Western Corporation
Simon & Schuster Building
Rockefeller Center
1230 Avenue of the Americas
New York, New York 10020

Library of Congress Cataloging in Publication Data

Main entry under title:

Looking good, feeling beautiful.

1.   Beauty, Personal.   2.   Cosmetics.
RA778.L863   646.7′2   80-11693

ISBN 25224-0

Illustrations by David Croland
Models' clothes provided by Henri Bendel
SIMON AND SCHUSTER and colophon are trademarks of Simon & Schuster
Manufactured in the United States of America
Composition by Dix Typesetting
Color Separations by Offset Separations
Printed and bound by Kingsport Press
1 3 5 7 9 10 8 6 4 2

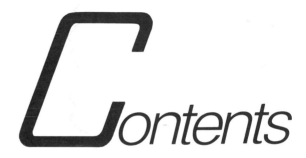

Contents

Introduction

To enjoy good health, to feel alive, and to look one's best are the goals of just about every woman I know. Although there was a period when many American women felt it was a bit self-indulgent to devote time and care to their looks, we know now that the desire to look good is both natural and healthy.

The urge to improve one's appearance is not new. For centuries people have done things to enhance their looks. Women of ancient Egypt, epitomized by Cleopatra, shadowed their eyes, tinted their nails, and treasured their wardrobe of scents. And who can forget the pictures of the women of the late 1700s with their tightly pinched waists, powdered pompadour hairdos, and bright lips?

But today enhancing one's looks is an individual matter. Rigid rules about beauty and fashion no longer apply. Designers do not dictate one silhouette to be worn by everyone, nor do beauty experts proclaim that you have to alter your eyebrows to conform to a universal shape.

Today's attractive woman is the one who selects what is particularly "right for her" from the many options available. Even fashion models reflect this attitude toward finding a personal style. I've attended photography sessions and seen them looking much like other attractive young women, without their makeup. But with makeup, as if by magic, each appears glamorously unique. Each has highlighted those features that make her special—high cheekbones, bright eyes, or full lips. A model needs to keep track of changing fashion looks, but most important she must discover her own special qualities and the techniques that can best emphasize them.

That is just what the Avon Beauty Book will help you do—learn about today's beauty trends and choose what is right for you. And because self-knowledge is so fundamental to good looks, our program begins in Chapter I with a Beauty Checkup, an act of self-assessment and self-discovery.

It's a good idea to give yourself such a checkup at least once a year. Like all living things, we are constantly changing, and so are our attitudes about what is attractive. The *lipstick shade or the hairstyle that you felt was so flattering a few years ago may do nothing for you now.*

As you start your program, keep in mind that making changes in your appearance will mean altering some of your habits and attitudes. That's not always easy or comfortable, but remember being in a rut is boring for you as well as those around you, and only change can lift you out of it.

"All right," you may be thinking, "I'm ready for self-discovery and I'm willing to make adjustments. But how do I find my personal style? How do I know what's right for me?" We believe this book can help you answer these questions.

As the world's largest beauty company with over a million Representatives worldwide, Avon is repeatedly asked for beauty advice.

Like the majority of women today, Avon Representatives and their customers lead demanding, busy lives. They want information that is basic, reliable, and practical. That is why we've approached the subject of beauty simply and directed you toward a look and attitude that we call "naturalness with style."

It's all here, gleaned from our beauty experts, cosmetologists, scientists, and consultants, and supplemented with proven tips and suggestions from women just like you. And because we believe that good looks and good health go hand in hand, we've taken care to include exercise, relaxation, and diet in your total beauty plan.

Making the commitment to become the most attractive woman you can be is really the biggest step. Once taken, you'll soon know that making some changes and investing some time in yourself is well worth it. It's not only looking good. It's feeling beautiful . . . every day of your life.

Phyllis B. Davis

*Group Vice President,
Avon Products, Inc.*

LOOKING GOOD, FEELING BEAUTIFUL

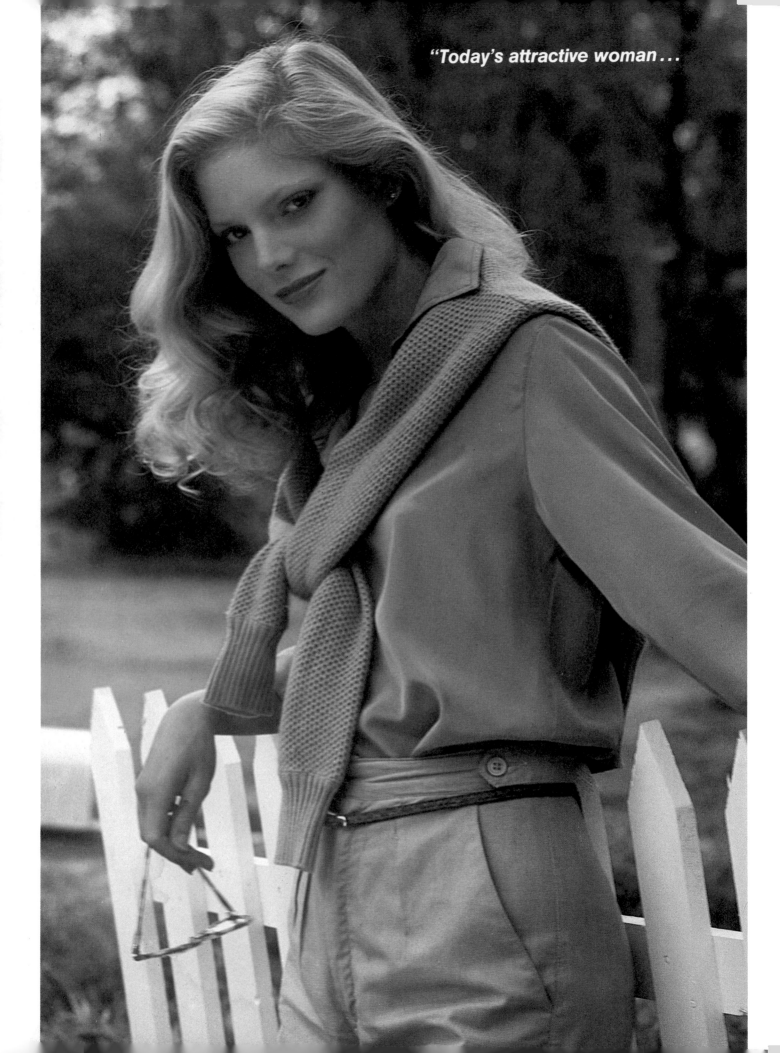

"Today's attractive woman...

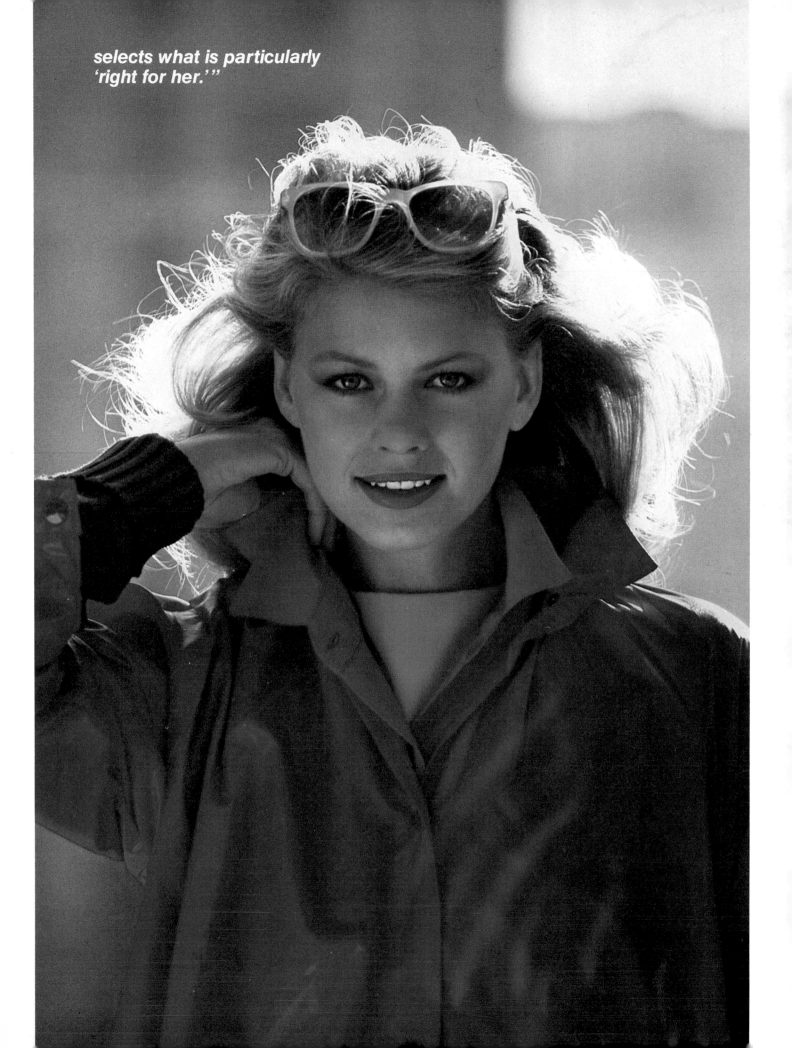

selects what is particularly
'right for her.'"

Step into a beautiful new life

What would it take to spark your looks from good to terrific? Probably far less than you think. Often a woman needs only to make a minor readjustment in the way she looks at herself to effect a major transformation.

The difficult part is taking a long, hard (but friendly!) look at yourself. Self-appraisal is never easy. We all tend to be severely critical of ourselves, acutely aware of fancied shortcomings, and often overlook features and characteristics that others find attractive. But an honest sizing up of the way you look today is a must; and with an attractive future in mind, such a cold, hard look can even be fairly pleasant.

Think of this as a Beauty Checkup. Just as you would see the doctor once or twice a year for an appraisal of the state of your health, schedule yourself for a private review of the state of your figure, your skin, your hair and nails. Set aside a quiet, unhurried time and run a warm, fragrant bath. Just after a relaxing bath is the time every woman looks and feels her prettiest: she is most feminine when she's still damp and glowing from the tub.

Before the bath, assemble the accessories you will need for your self-appraisal session: a tape measure for accurate and up-to-date figure data . . . a bathroom scale . . . two or three mirrors—ideally, a full-length mirror and a hand-held mirror as well as a magnifying mirror. And be sure to have handy a pencil or pen and a Beauty Notebook. To set the mood and attitude for a Beauty Checkup, you might want to be lulled by music as you relax in the bath. Tune a transistor radio to a station with few commercials and lots of beautiful music. Don't forget to add some sweet-smelling, skin-softening bath oil to the tub. It's good for your skin and your spirit. Allow yourself ten minutes of soaking in the warm, fragrant water before blotting yourself dry and beginning your self-analysis.

Stand before the full-length mirror to study yourself from head to toe. Use the hand-held mirror along with the large mirror so that you can see rear and profile views. Study yourself as you are today. Look at the woman who's there now—not the woman you were five or ten years ago, or six months ago. We are all changing every day.

Take time to study everything about yourself, and make notes on your findings from head to toe. Look at your face. Are your eyebrows straggly? Would a little more exercise or more sleep perk up your complexion? Look at your hair. Is it a bit lackluster this week? Are you due for a great new cut? Look at your arms. Would some spot exercising help tone the flabby flesh of your upper arms? Or are they looking good? Look at your body. Is your waist a shade roly-poly? How about your hips? Perhaps you're used to being told that you have beautiful legs. Look at them. Are they still terrific, or would some running help trim the upper thighs? Look at your hands. Is your nail enamel chipped? Look at your feet. Are they pampered enough to be on display in winter as well as in summer?

Are you thoroughly depressed after studying the state of your looks? Don't be. Some things can be helped by diet and exercise. Other things can be corrected by beauty techniques, and we'll talk about all of those. But for the moment, how about some instant remedies?

THE IMPORTANCE OF POSTURE

Would you like a slimmer waist? Immediately? That's easy.

Stand in a comfortable position before a full-length mirror. Look at yourself, then close your eyes. Now imagine that there is a big pink balloon, helium-filled, attached to the top of your head. Concentrate on the balloon, relax and let your body go limp. Let the shiny balloon lift you up until your feet barely touch the floor. Relax as the balloon floats up to the ceiling; it will pull your body up with it, stretching the spinal cord, which has the effect of lifting your spine and your chest—but let your arms and shoulders hang down freely and comfortably as a puppet's while your neck is lifting up and away from the body. Now that you're comfortably held aloft by your beautiful balloon, open your eyes. Doesn't your waist (your whole body, in fact) look slimmer? Don't you look a little bit taller, better? That's good posture.

It's the easiest beauty tool of all. But most of us don't know how to make use of it. Most people assume a rigid uncomfortable position at the very mention of the word "posture." Their backs arch; their shoulders are hunched up and jerked back awkwardly. It looks as uncomfortable as it feels. This sort of rigid stance is an insult to the body, yet most people feel that it is what's meant by good posture.

Correct posture is a simple matter of letting the bones align themselves naturally. It's the easiest favor you can do yourself. Your build and your bones are a result of genetics, and their shape determines yours for life. But your carriage can make the structure of your body seem more nearly ideal.

"... An honest sizing up of the way you look today is a must."

The way you carry yourself can even determine whether you appear energetic or tired, optimistic or pessimistic, younger or older. Dr. Leroy Perry, a sports chiropractor and nutritionist in Los Angeles, says, "There's no secret to the fountain of youth. It's posture." When you are tired and just drooping along, you need only say to yourself, "My balloon is dragging" to remind yourself to stand up straight.

Here's another mental exercise for posture. It's one dancers sometimes use—and you know how beautifully dancers carry themselves.

Stand comfortably and imagine that it is possible to slip a tiny air pillow for comfort between each two vertebrae in your lower back. There are five vertebrae between the sacroiliac and the rib cage. Concentrate on separating each one in turn just a little farther from the next, giving them a little more "breathing space." Focus your attention on each one, as if you were opening and extending the distance between pelvis and rib cage. Breathe deeply as you lift, and you will feel more comfortable and relaxed immediately. That slight extra space in your middle allows the internal organs to expand and to function more smoothly than they can in a pinched position.

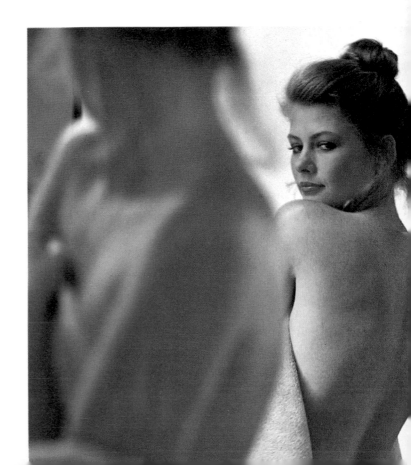

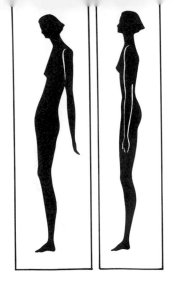

"The way you carry yourself can even determine whether you appear energetic or tired, optimistic or pessimistic, younger or older."

Your shoulders are the only part of your body that should not lift in the process. When everything else is Up, shoulders stay Down. Shoulders should always be parallel to the floor, while everything else aims for the ceiling.

Just to make sure your body gets the right idea, try this: Place your right hand, fingers spread and palm flat, on your right shoulder. Place the left hand on the left shoulder. Slowly swing your elbows down close to your body and try to touch them to your waist. Of course, they won't quite touch, but your shoulders will be in proper alignment.

Do this exercise in the morning, then from time to time during the day when you think of it. Also practice lifting your arms while keeping your shoulders down. Within a few days you won't need these little posture checks, because proper carriage will become an easy, habitual condition. But just at first, do all the posture-improving memory tricks every morning as you check your appearance in the mirror before starting the day. Smile, and memorize the way you are carrying your body and the way you look right now. It will help keep your spirits—and your balloon—lifted.

Improved posture just naturally leads the way to better breathing.

The tensions of modern-day living tend to promote shallow, irregular breathing. Since breath control is an automatic body function, you needn't worry about staying alive with that kind of breathing. But if you want to look and feel glad to be alive, that's a different matter. Then you need to take a few deep, cleansing breaths from time to time.

Dr. Kenneth H. Cooper, the man who devised aerobics (exercises that are aimed at increasing cardiovascular efficiency) says, "If you don't breathe deeply from time to time, properly ventilating your lungs, you could end up with a collapse of the lungs' periphery. Also, the exercise strengthens the muscles that support the rib cage."

Besides, deep breathing improves sluggish circulation to help your skin look fresher and the whites of your eyes brighter. When you feel groggy, breathing exercises can snap you into a fresh, alert state of mind. When you feel tense, concentrating on your breathing can be a wonderful natural tranquilizer.

Here is a Yoga recipe for deep, cleansing breathing: Inhale through the nostrils as deeply as you can, really sucking air down into the abdomen. Let your stomach and diaphragm swell to accommodate the air. You want to fill the cavity with pure, fresh oxygen. Now slowly contract your stomach, all the way up from the pelvis to the rib cage. (At first, while learning the movement, use your fingers to press your abdomen in and up.) Force all the air up from your stomach and out through your open mouth. Repeat three times.

This slow, controlled breathing is easy, effective and unobtrusive. Next time you feel yourself tensing up out of boredom or frustration, try this breathing exercise and see how much calmer and more alert you soon feel.

REMINDERS FOR INSTANT BEAUTY

■ Your bones are light—only about one-fifth of total body weight. Carry them that way.

■ Crossing your legs is not necessarily bad for you, no matter what you have been told. There is a right and a wrong way. The healthy way is to cross legs high (when you are wearing pants or you are alone), with the ankle of one leg resting on the knee of the supporting leg. The wrong way is with legs pressed so tightly together as to constrict circulation. It's even worse if you pretzel one foot around the other leg.

14

■ Actresses learn to use movements and gestures to appear older or younger. So can you. Here's a sampling to practice with. . . .

Walking: Young Way—Head back, spine straight, arms swinging at sides. **Old Way**—Head jutting forward, shoulders slumped, arms up and in as if to clutch stomach.

Standing: Young Way—Knees slightly flexed, feet fairly close together. **Old Way**—Knees locked, feet wide apart.

Making Up: Young Way—Head back and high, looking down your nose into the mirror. **Old Way**—Neck craning closer to the mirror.

■ Have groceries loaded into two bags rather than one if you will be carrying them. For best body balance, always carry an equal weight on either side. If you must carry a single heavy suitcase or grocery bag, switch it from side to side frequently.

■ If your kitchen sink is too high for you to stand and work at comfortably, sit on a stool that puts you at a comfortable height. It's better for your back, your legs, your whole body. The ideal solution, of course, would be to have the sink and the counter height in your kitchen altered to suit you. It might not be such an expensive project as you think, and the results will improve your life immeasurably.

■ Sit on the edge of your chair. Weight thus rests on the bones at the lower edge of the pelvis. This helps strengthen the back and helps to control fanny spread.

■ When seated at your desk, keep one foot flat on the floor and elevate the other by propping it up on a thick telephone directory, a small box or a firm pillow. Alternate from time to time. This is a real help to circulation.

■ Keep your chin up and your head will follow. You'll prevent a double chin if you hold your head high and don't let your chin drop when you turn to look back over your shoulder.

■ To aid circulation, sit on the floor when you are relaxing. When your legs are level your body doesn't have to work so hard to pump the blood up, particularly if the veins aren't being pressed by the edge of a chair. You also look more graceful sitting down on the floor if your spine is erect, weight resting on the pelvis; legs are up with knees bent and hands are clasped lightly over the ankles.

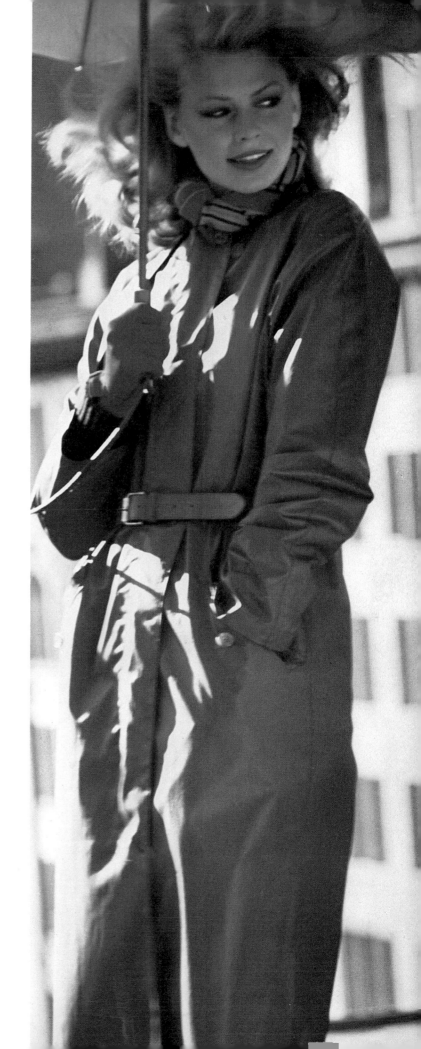

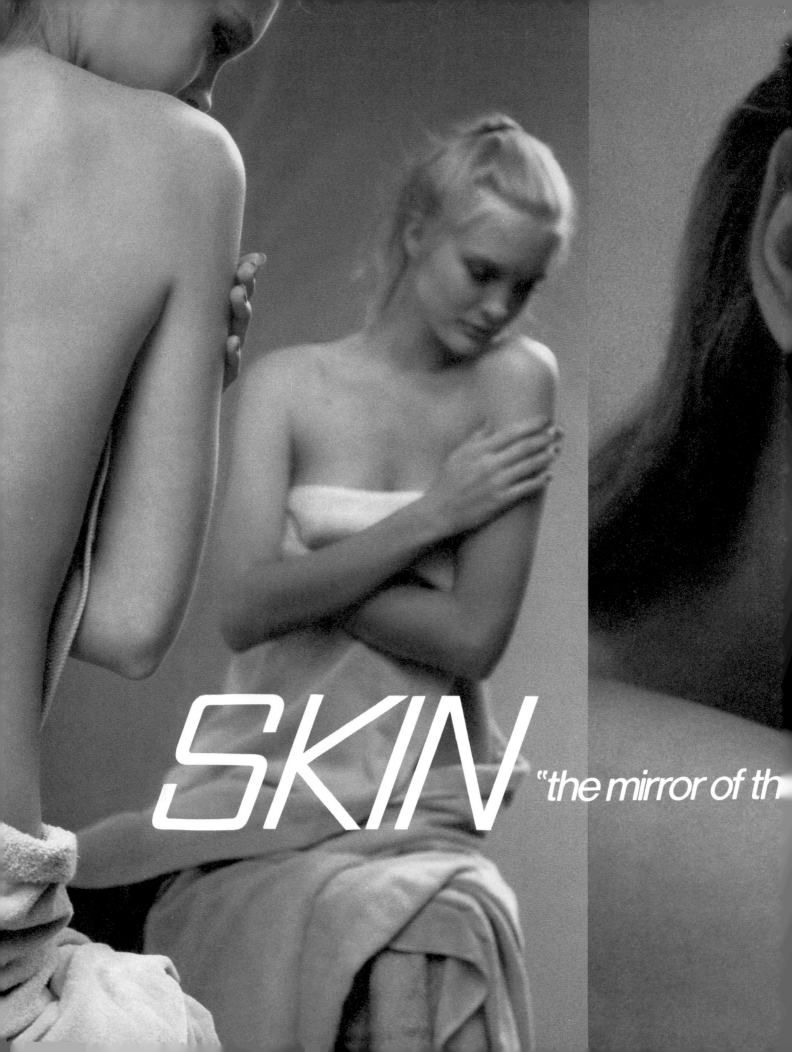

SKIN

"the mirror of th

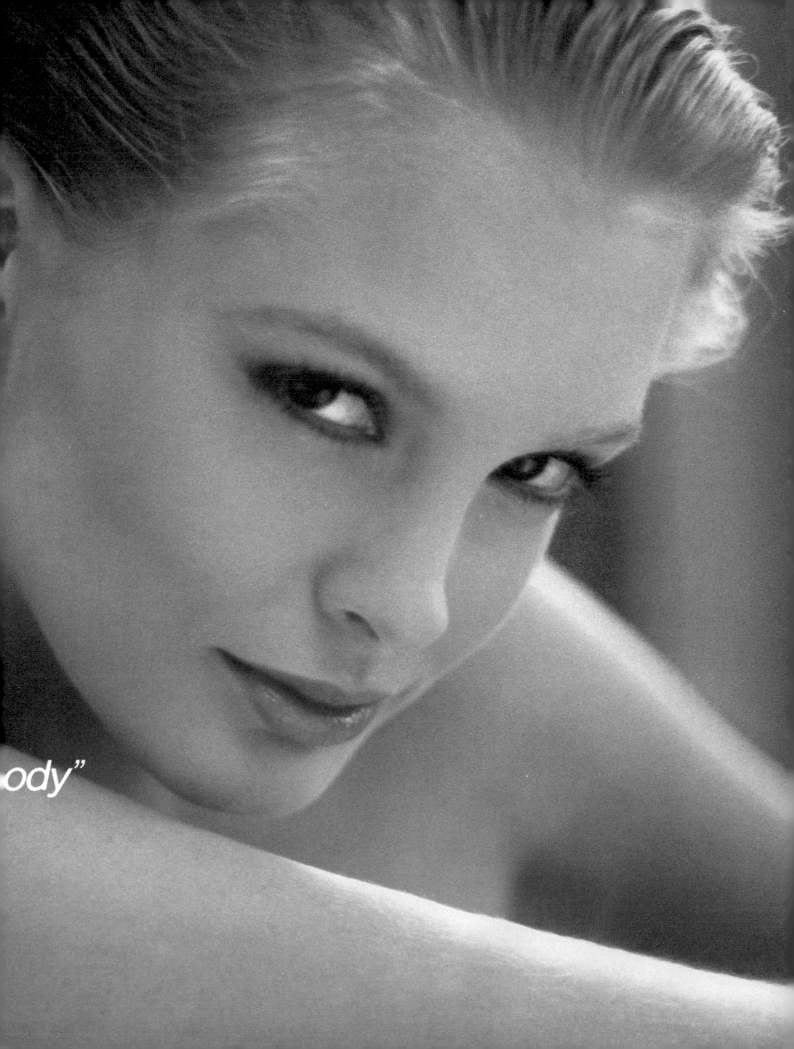

ody"

Give yourself the best-looking skin

You write your own life story every day, and your skin is where others read it. Skin has been called the mirror of the body. It accurately reflects the state of your health, past and present. But you can rewrite the script, because skin is constantly renewing itself.

New cells mature in approximately fifteen days, and old skin cells are constantly being shed. Skin responds almost overnight to a new program of proper cleansing and care.

We'll get to specifics in a minute. First, though, you should familiarize yourself with your own wonderful wrapping.

"Skin responds almost overnight to a new program aimed at clearing away past neglect . . ."

SKIN IS:

The largest organ of your body, as important for life as the heart. Skin accounts for about 15 percent of your total weight.

Only about four one-hundredths of one inch thick over most of the body. It's thicker, and ridged for traction, on the palms and on the soles of the feet. It's much thinner on the eyelids.

Defensive armor for the body. It prevents outside attacks on the body by microbes and injuries, even manufactures its own antiseptic —the clear fluid called lymph. The skin also prevents the escape of vital fluids from within the body.

A complex relay center for messages to and from the brain. Sensory-nerve endings within the skin record pleasure and pain, heat and cold, and other conditions currently affecting the body, and transmit this news to the brain, which then signals motor-nerve endings in the skin. These nerve endings trigger the muscle and gland functions causing perspiration, shivering, gooseflesh, and blushing.

A major body temperature regulator, as well as a ventilation/purification system for the body. Skin helps keep the body's internal temperature at a constant 98.6° F. (37° C.). Sebum helps lubricate the skin, and perspiration aids in temperature control and flushing away impurities. Sweat glands open to the skin surface through millions of pores all over the body and transmit cooling perspiration to the surface. Oily sebum, to lubricate skin and skin and keep it supple, is secreted by sebaceous glands at the base of tiny hairs which cover the body.

THERE'S MORE TO SKIN THAN MEETS THE EYE

Thin as it is, the skin is composed of two individual layers, plus a third layer of fatty tissue just beneath the skin. The top layer, the epidermis, is composed at its surface of flattened cells of keratin which are constantly being sloughed off and replaced. Within the epidermis are specialized cells, called melanocytes, which produce melanin, the pigment that gives skin (and hair) its color. When the skin is exposed to the sun, melanin production is increased and a tan results.

Below the epidermis, but bound to it, is the skin's second layer, the dermis. Collagen and elastin, the major proteins in skin, are produced in the dermis. They knit together to form skin that has a supple, elastic tone and strength. Glands and tiny blood vessels in the dermis nourish the skin, hair and nails, and supply the fluids that lubricate and protect the epidermis. The dermis houses capillaries, perspiration glands and hair roots. Beneath the dermis is the subcutaneous fatty tissue, which is thicker in some places than in others. Its "hills and valleys" are what help determine the contours of the face.

"Too high an acid level can create problems of itchy skin and scalp, and a cleanser that is too acid just won't clean."

Healthy skin constantly secretes water (perspiration) and an oily material (sebum) which emulsify on the surface of the skin into a single substance that lubricates and protects. This emulsion makes the skin look plump and moist, and when skin and its surroundings are operating under peak conditions, it is chemically balanced to provide an antiseptic condition that kills microbes on the skin surface.

Many years ago, the chemist Marchionini researched the chemical structure of this natural skin lubrication. He used the pH scale. This scale goes from 0 to 14. Low numbers indicate acid materials, high numbers alkaline ones. Neutral, neither acid nor alkaline, is pH 7. Marchionini's studies showed that a range from pH 3.0 to pH 5.5 occurs on healthy skin. He reasoned that this microscopic film of acidic moisture over the skin and hair was a kind of protective covering, which he called the "acid mantle."

Today we know that the skin is quickly adaptable and much more resilient and self-protective than was once supposed. You needn't worry about the natural acid mantle of your skin, so long as you keep your system functioning in a normal, healthy state and use mild, gentle products to clean skin and hair. Of course, you wouldn't wash your face or your hair with laundry soap, which is full of free alkali. But don't try to find a very acidic cleanser, either. Too high an acid level can create problems of itchy skin and scalp, and a cleanser that is too acid just won't clean. In hard water especially, an acid solution will "complex" (solidify) dirt and grease on the skin so they cannot be rinsed away. Then, in a short time, the skin is as dirty as before washing. A cleanser that is too acid is easy to spot: it won't lather. Cleansers don't normally lather until they are at least pH 7—neutral. A nearly neutral to slightly alkaline cleanser, well rinsed, is best for your skin.

Most soaps and cleansers made for facial use are either close to neutral or slightly alkaline. Rinse thoroughly (warm, not hot, water is best for skin). Skin is instantly returned to its pre-

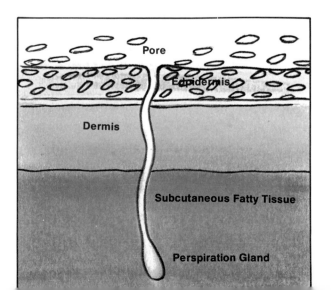

Pore

Epidermis

Dermis

Subcutaneous Fatty Tissue

Perspiration Gland

ferred state of acidity if, after cleansing, you use an astringent toner. Toners, and most other products for after-cleansing skin care, are formulated to fall within the range of pH 4.5 to pH 5.5—ideal for beautiful healthy skin.

SKIN IS MOISTURE

Specifically, water. Healthy skin is up to 90 percent water. Think of the words to describe pretty skin—"moist," "dewy." Water trapped within the cells keeps skin plumped and firm. Water keeps skin extended to the utmost, so that it looks almost transparent and unlined.

But the body, and the skin, lose water constantly in order to stay healthy. Breathing, you exhale water. On an average day, through elimination and perspiration, the body eliminates more than 1½ pints of water. Without skin to act as a water barrier, your body would simply dry up. In disease, and conditions of dehydration, the body loses so much water that it shrinks slightly. Skin then contracts, becoming slightly more opaque and slightly more wrinkled.

How can you prevent this? "Just add water." Doctors say you should drink six to eight glasses a day. If you find plain water lacking in appeal, drink sparkling mineral water with a slice of lime. Or try adding just a little splash of fruit juice to still or sparkling water. (If you are watching your salt intake, get a sparkling spring water or seltzer. Most club soda has added salt.) A favorite health spa treat is to fill a beautiful crystal goblet with iced sparkling spring water topped with one tablespoon of natural apple juice. It looks like champagne, and it tastes delicious. There are a number of other delicious, low-calorie ways to make drinking water seem more festive and satisfying—iced peppermint tea and a tall glass of pink rose-hips tea over ice are only two of the possibilities using herb teas from the health-foods counter of the supermarket. But don't add honey or sugar and fruit. The more you add to the glass the less water it holds, and the less thirst-quenching it becomes.

"Who has time for a regimen when she has to get the kids off to school and be at work on time?"

Doctors have rated the thirst-quenching ability of various drinks. Only water scores 100 percent.

You might be more inclined to drink the water your skin needs if you drink it from a beautiful glass. If you want to feel like a pampered princess, drink water from a crystal goblet. Check the closeouts corner of your department store. A single goblet of a discontinued pattern or broken set can usually be found for very little.

Water inside keeps skin plump and glowing. Oddly enough, water on the surface of the skin encourages dryness.

For the best-looking skin, you must trap water within the upper layer of the skin, yet keep water off the surface of the skin. For this double task, a protective lubricant or moisturizer is needed. The skin manufactures sebum to cover the skin surface with an invisible, water-repellent shield. But in this world of artificial heating and cooling, of exposure to parching sun and wind, sebum is insufficient. For attractive healthy skin a good moisturizer for the face and a good moisturizing lotion for the hands and body are vital. Most moisturizers contain both humectants and emollients. Humectants attract water within the tissues and draw it to the cells of the epidermis to keep this top layer of skin plump and hydrated. Emol-

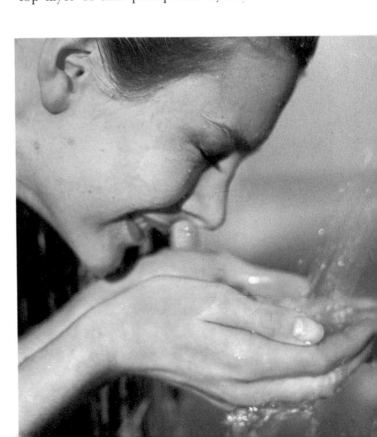

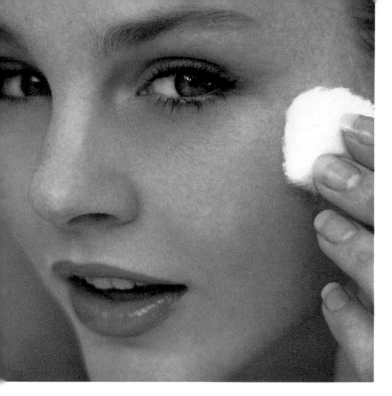

This can be done with special creams called exfoliating creams or with an abrasive cleansing puff. The abrasive cleansing puff is designed to be used with rinse-off cleansers or with soap and water to give the face a very minor form of the epidermabrasion favored by dermatologists. It will not only make your face feel cleaner, but it will also look cleaner as well.

Work up to it. If you've always creamed your face to cleanse, then use your cleansing cream on a wet washcloth and scrub. Unless skin is extra dry, extra sensitive, you can graduate within a day or two to the cleansing puff. Use it in quick, light circular motions on wet skin along with a mild soap. You will probably be delighted with the results of this brisk cell sloughing.

lients coat the skin with a lubricating shield, to help prevent the evaporation of moisture which has been trapped in the upper layer of the skin.

NO TIME FOR A REGIMEN?

You hear a lot about programs and regimens of skin care. It sounds forbidding, doesn't it? Who has time for a regimen when she has to get the kids off to school and be at work on time?

Well, a regimen can be just the simple 1-2-3 of cleanse-tone-moisturize. People in the beauty business decided that "your skin regimen" sounded a little prettier than "how to clean your face." Just do the good things and don't be put off by the words. It's quicker to do than to describe.

EVERY SKIN NEEDS
A GOOD CLEANSING

Most of the dead cells the skin constantly sheds just fall off and fly away unseen—left behind on the pillow, rinsed off in the bath, shed as we go about the day. Most of them. But not all. A lot of those dead cells remain on the surface of your skin and hide the fresh new skin beneath. Black women are very much aware of this and know the condition as ashiness.

You have to scrub away the clinging dead cells in order to reveal younger, fresher skin.

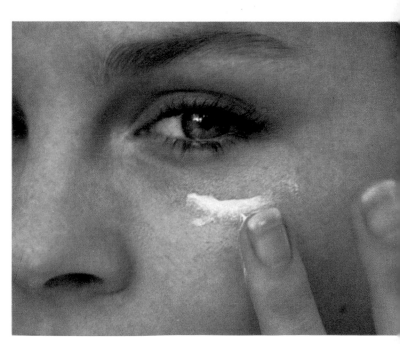

"For the best looking skin use moisturizer regularly to coat the skin with a lubricating shield."

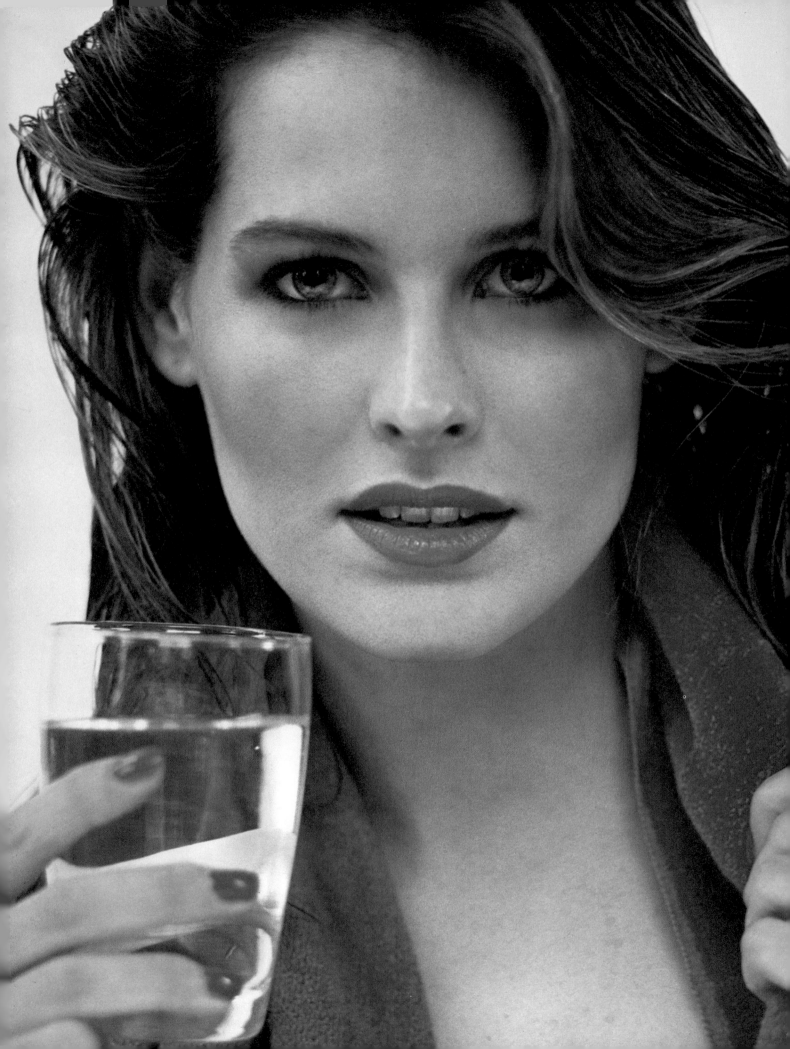

If your skin is Dry

If your pores are almost invisible . . . if your skin never or seldom breaks out . . . if your skin is flaky, sometimes itchy . . . if your face doesn't really get shiny during the day after you make up in the morning . . . if you can go four days at least before your hair gets sticky between shampoos . . . your skin is dry.

SPECIAL NOTE: Neglect shows fast in the form of crepiness, so be generous with protective measures. Be gentle but vigilant about sloughing off dry dead cells that dull the surface beauty.

P.M.

Evening first—that's when dry skin should get a thorough cleansing.

WHAT TO USE	HOW TO USE IT
1. Dry-skin cleanser:	Massage with fingertips upward and outward from throat.
Tissue-off type	Dampen a tissue to remove all traces of makeup and cleanser.
or	
Rinse-off cleanser or cleansing bar	Scrub face lightly using wet washcloth or abrasive puff with rinse-off cleanser or bar. Rinse thoroughly with cool to lukewarm water.
2. Low-alcohol skin toner	Apply with a cotton pad to erase any remaining bit of makeup, cream, or soap.
3. Rich night cream	Protect your skin with a thin film of cream. Apply 15 minutes before bed, then blot off any excess.

A.M.

An abbreviated version of the evening routine because you are not removing dirt and makeup. Also, dry skin does not secrete as much oil.

WHAT TO USE	HOW TO USE IT
1. Low-alcohol skin toner	Splash your face with lukewarm water and then cool water before applying toner on a cotton pad. Blot face dry.
2. Moisturizer	Rub a little moisturizer between your fingers—body heat liquefies cream so it spreads easily and goes farther—and sweep it up lightly from base of throat to hairline. Blot off excess.

WEEKLY

WHAT TO USE	HOW TO USE IT
1. Peel-off mask and/or 2. Moisturizing mask	Use a deep-cleansing peel-off mask alone or followed with a second mask to moisturize skin. Always apply a thin film of moisturizer to very dry skin before using a peel-off mask.

If your skin is Oily

If your pores are very obvious . . . if your skin breaks out often . . . if your face is shiny most of the time or gets shiny within a couple of hours after making up . . . if you must shampoo daily to prevent your hair from looking and feeling sticky . . . you have oily skin.

SPECIAL NOTE: Your skin demands a lot of care and may seem the most troublesome type, but in the long run, oily skin is a blessing. Skin usually becomes drier with age, so the young woman with oily skin becomes the woman whose skin is moist and less lined late in life.

A.M.

Morning first, because oily skin secretes oils during the night. You should start with a thorough cleansing.

WHAT TO USE	HOW TO USE IT
1. Cleanser designed for oily skin	If skin is troubled with acne, use specially designed products; if acne is a chronic problem, follow your doctor's advice. The gentle use of a cleansing puff with an abrasive surface helps keep clogged pores open, as well as removing excess oil and shine. Rinse with lukewarm water. Blot dry.
2. Astringent	Saturate a cotton pad with astringent and wipe upward and outward. Repeat until pad is clean.
3. A light moisturizer	Unless your skin is very oily, moisturizer will help protect it, especially the eye, cheek and throat areas.

AFTERNOON

WHAT TO USE	HOW TO USE IT
Cleanser, astringent, and light moisturizer	Refresh by removing makeup, cleansing, and toning. Follow with a light moisturizer and fresh makeup, if you wish.

P.M.

WHAT TO USE	HOW TO USE IT
1. Cleanser	As in the morning and afternoon.
2. Astringent	As in the morning and afternoon.
3. Moisturizer	Only around the eyes.

WEEKLY

WHAT TO USE	HOW TO USE IT
1. Clay-based deep-cleansing mask or peel-off mask	Add a facial mask to the nice things that you do for yourself on your Beauty Time. Use either type of facial mask listed to give oily skin a thorough cleansing.

If your skin is a Combination

If your pores are visible . . . if your skin breaks out in a monthly cycle or very infrequently . . . if your skin becomes shiny in the early afternoon when you make up in the morning . . . if your face is oily in the T-zone (forehead, nose and chin) . . . if you can wait three or four days between shampoos . . . your skin is a combination type.

SPECIAL NOTE: If you are fortunate enough to have that delicately balanced skin between Dry and Oily, yours is the rare type called Normal. You should use products designed for normal skin to maintain this condition.

P.M.
Evening first, because that's when combination skin gets a thorough, scrupulous cleansing.

WHAT TO USE	HOW TO USE IT
1. Cleanser: Tissue-off type	Massage with fingertips upward and outward from throat. Dampen a tissue to remove all traces of makeup and cleanser.
or	
Rinse-off cleanser or cleansing bar	Scrub face lightly using wet washcloth or abrasive puff with rinse-off cleanser or bar. Rinse thoroughly with cool to lukewarm water.
2. Astringent and mild toner	Use astringent for oily areas and toner for dry areas. Saturate cotton pads and wipe until pads are clean.
3. Night cream	Apply only to delicate dry areas, such as eyes, cheeks and throat, for protection while you sleep.

A.M.
A quick, abbreviated version of the evening routine.

WHAT TO USE	HOW TO USE IT
1. Cleanser	Cleanse only those areas of your face that become shiny overnight. Rinse with cool water.
2. Astringent and mild toner	As in the evening.
3. Moisturizer	Moisturize lightly from throat to hairline, covering all but the oiliest areas.

WEEKLY

WHAT TO USE	HOW TO USE IT
1. A facial mask	You can use a deep-cleansing mask on oily areas and a moisturizing one on the dry areas.

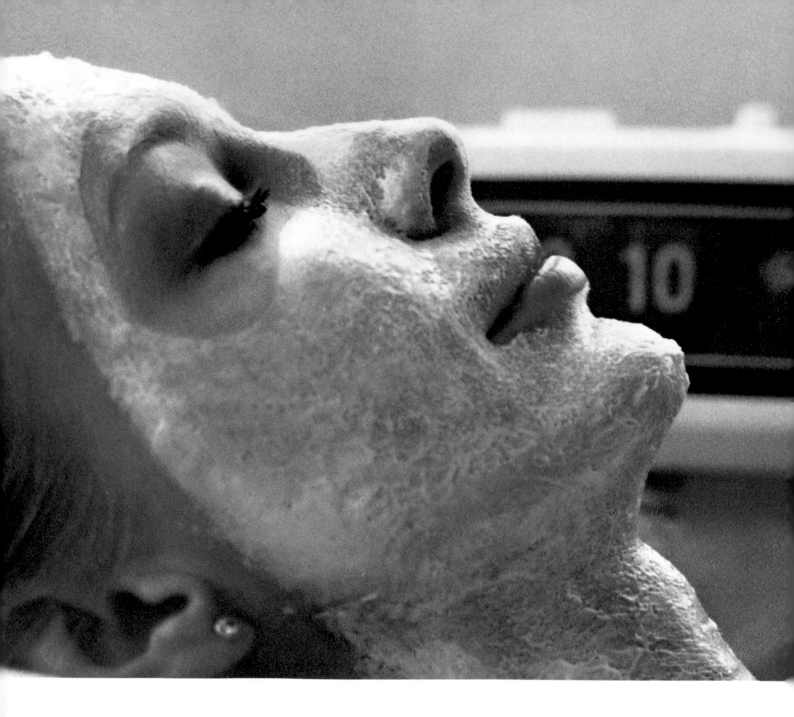

EVERY SKIN TYPE RESPONDS TO A TREAT

The Beautiful People we read about always seem to be going off to facial salons and spas where wonderful things are done to their skin. Just getting away from the pressures of a job and a family for a quickie vacation would do wonderful things for our skin, too. Few of us have the leisure time or money for visits to skin-care salons. But we can all try to squeeze in an hour sometime during the week for a mini-vacation for the skin.

Before proceeding with your skin treat, prepare an atmosphere of total comfort in which to relax later. Put on some soothing music at low volume. Pick a cozy spot where you can stretch out with your feet propped up higher than your head. Pile up a few pillows for the purpose. Have an alarm clock or kitchen timer handy.

Now, before you get comfortable, have a gentle, cleansing facial vapor bath. Heat water in a large, shallow saucepan on the stove. Toss a bag of chamomile herb tea into the water when it starts to simmer. (The herb is optional, but does give the vapors a soothing, delicious aroma. You can find chamomile herb teabags in the health-foods area of the supermarket or at natural-food shops.)

26

"Few of us have the leisure time or money for visits to skin-care salons. But we can all try to squeeze in an hour sometime during the week for a mini-vacation for the skin."

Take the steaming pan off the burner. Use a towel over your head to make a sort of tent arrangement and bend over the pan. The towel prevents the steam from escaping. Close your eyes and let the warm vapors play across your face. In the moist warmth, pores throw off impurities, and your skin will be quite clean by the time the water stops steaming. Lift your head, blot your face with the towel and use your fingertips to apply a facial mask. (Refer to the Care Chart for the best kinds of masks for your skin type.)

Read the directions carefully. Cover forehead, nose and chin with the mask. Avoid eyes, lips and hairline. Stroke mask back from cheeks to the ears. Check the specified time, and set the alarm or a kitchen timer. Don't leave a mask on longer than the directed time; it doesn't increase the mask's benefits to skin, and removal takes longer.

While the mask is working, just lie back and relax to music. Later, if you've chosen to follow with a second mask, set the timer again and relax a bit more. This is a blissful vacation for the skin, one from which it returns with a lasting glow.

When applying a peel-off facial mask, be sure to avoid the sensitive eye, nose and mouth areas and the hairline. When removing the mask, begin at the forehead and gently work down with both hands so that the mask comes off in one piece.

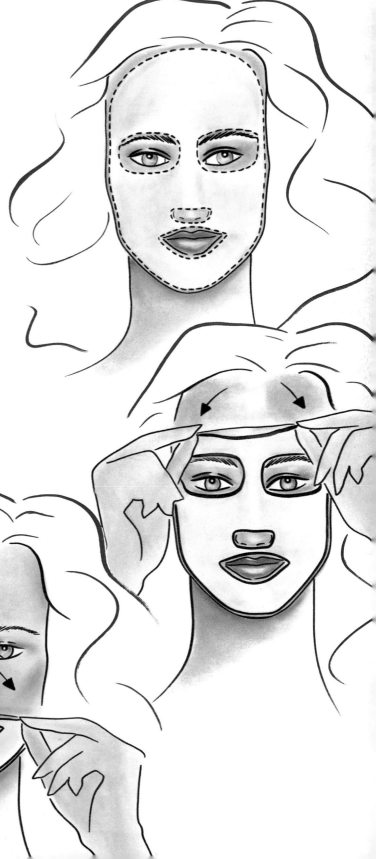

Even with the most loving care...

Even with the most loving care, skin sometimes falls victim to a problem. Some of the most common skin vexations are listed below. Some respond right away to a little special attention at home. But others don't. Stubborn ones, including those caused by allergies, can't be solved alone. Turn them over to your family doctor or a dermatologist.

Dermatologists spend their lives studying the skin and its health. Remember, skin acts as an early-warning signal for many internal illnesses. Seeing a dermatologist for what seems a little problem may spare you larger ones. You really owe it to yourself to find a good dermatologist if your skin takes a puzzling turn for the worse.

Ask your family doctor or the county medical society for a good skin specialist. Or check the local hospital. Some dermatological clinics at university-affiliated hospitals provide almost-free treatment.

ACNE: Almost 90 percent of all adolescents, and quite a large number of adults, suffer from acne to some degree. Having lots of company doesn't ease the misery, though. It may help to know that acne doesn't strike just because you fail to keep your skin clean, or because you eat chocolate. Glandular and hormonal activity are usually behind acne. Puberty brings an increase both in the activity of the sebaceous glands and in hormonal production. Both male hormones —androgens—and female hormones—estrogens—are produced by both sexes. The hormones are accepted or rejected by receptors in our cells. Cellular receptors in some people are more receptive to the male hormones, androgens. For these people, acne is likely to develop. Just how and why the androgens trigger greater sebaceous-gland activity is not entirely understood. But doctors do know what to do about it. Real breakthroughs have been reported recently. Several new drugs have been found to relieve or cure even very severe cases that did not respond to previous therapy. Currently, tetracycline therapy is beneficial for many patients. Dermatologists can sometimes trace adult acne to such diverse causes as cough medicines, diet pills and birth-control pills. But most foods are off the list of culprits suspected of causing acne. If you find that a specific food triggers a breakout, avoid it. The foods you might be careful of are those containing iodides: artichokes, spinach, peanuts, sea salt, shellfish, saltwater fish. Otherwise, eat a wide variety of foods and stop worrying. Stress isn't good for anything, and it's very bad for acne.

In many cases, acne can be treated with non-prescription soaps and lotions. Effective ones will contain one or more of the following ingredients: benzoyl peroxide, precipitated sulfur, salicylic acid, resorcinol. Use the treatment as directed, and use special acne-formula products to cleanse and to cover and treat blemishes.

Wash your face as frequently as convenient to help eliminate excess oils. Plenty of fresh-air exercise is helpful. Increased circulation brought about by exercise aids in healing acne blemishes.

BLACKHEADS: A blackhead is a clogged oil gland. The opening of the gland is blocked by excess sebum. When the sebum is exposed to air it oxidizes, thus darkens, and the blackhead, or comedo, is formed. Use a facial sauna, or heat a saucepan of water until it simmers. Remove the pan from the heat and hold your face in the steam, with a towel tented over your head to hold the steam in. Then apply a peel-off or clay-based facial mask to draw them out. Follow with astringent toner. Don't squeeze. You risk infection and damaging the skin.

WHITEHEADS: A whitehead is composed of hardened, fatty materials that collect below the surface of the skin in the opening of the oil glands. If consistent, thorough cleansing according to your skin type does not help whiteheads disappear, a dermatologist can remove them. Do not squeeze: the whiteheads won't come out, and you risk infection.

HIVES: A case of hives can be an allergic reaction, and it can also be brought on by stress. Many medications—even one as simple as aspirin—can aggravate hives. See the dermatologist.

SPIDERY RED LINES: The technical name for these tiny broken capillaries is telangiecteses. They usually appear around the nose and on the cheeks. Heredity can predispose you to them; exposing the skin to extreme weather can cause them, as can using very hot water on the skin, and immoderate use of alcohol. You can cover them with foundation, or have them removed safely by a dermatologist.

FRECKLES: Freckles are simply little isolated islands of melanin in the skin. The sun seems to intensify them, although a tendency to freckle is hereditary. Attempts to remove them medically are futile, but some bleaching creams do help. Or you can cover them with makeup. Or best of all, stop worrying and recognize that to people who don't have them, freckles are charming.

RED PINHEAD SPOTS: Tiny dark-red spots on the skin may look like insect bites, but when they don't hurt or itch may be what dermatologists call cherry angioma. They appear on more than 75 percent of all men and women over thirty. They are harmless, but can be removed safely by a dermatologist.

MOLES: Moles should be let alone by you, but they may be removed by a dermatologist. Never tweeze a hair growing from a mole, although you can safely clip it short. Be sure to see your doctor should you notice any change in a mole's size or appearance.

STRETCH MARKS: These are ruptures of the collagen and elastin below the epidermis. They are sometimes triggered by rapid weight gain and loss. The most common periods for the formation of stretch marks are during pregnancies and during adolescence (particularly if the adolescent is overweight), both times of hormonal changes in the body. Stretch marks are often highly colored at first, but soon fade. What makes them even more noticeable, though, is the faint puckering of the skin over the stretch mark. Cover stick makeup can sometimes make stretch marks less apparent. Dermabrasion and plastic surgery are more radical (though not always successful) means of eliminating stretch marks.

SKIN TAGS: These are wartlike bumps, often on the neck. They are not dangerous and are thought to be hereditary, though they are sometimes caused by taking birth-control pills. A dermatologist can safely remove them.

ECZEMA: An inflammation of skin can be limited to a small portion of the body, or cover large areas. To soothe the pain and itching, cool compresses often help. See a dermatologist.

MASK OF PREGNANCY: The technical name for this discoloration of the skin, usually in a butterfly shape on the upper part of the face, is melasma or chloasma. Birth-control pills may be responsible. A bleaching cream can help remove it. Look for one containing 1.5 to 2 percent hydroquinone. This is the only active ingredient which is both safe and effective. Be careful out in the sun. After using a bleaching cream, avoid excessive exposure to sunlight or use a sunscreen.

SUN WARTS: These thickened, scaly, discolored spots on the skin are dangerous. They are precancerous and should be treated by a dermatologist. He uses a topical drug (5-Fluorouracil) or cryosurgery (freezing with liquid nitrogen) to remove them or he removes them surgically. The technical name for a sun wart is actinic keratosis, and they are commonly found on the back of the hands or on the face.

PSORIASIS: Patches of silvery-white scales over red, inflamed skin can occur anywhere on the body. Psoriasis is not contagious. It comes about when skin cells grow much too rapidly. It can be treated by a dermatologist. For information ask your doctor or write: National Psoriasis Foundation, Suite 200, 6415 South West Canyon Court, Portland, OR 97221.

AGING SKIN

This is, strictly speaking, an overall skin condition rather than a specific problem. But it is *the* big skin worry, the one that will affect us all, and in many different forms. Wrinkles, crepy skin, sagging, skin blotching and darkening—the list of symptoms of aging skin is long, and every item on it is vexing.

There are measures to take, however, that will help prevent, arrest, correct or at the very least minimize the apparent effects of aging skin. The first step in winning the war is to know your enemy.

THE SIGNS OF AGING SKIN
(and some first-aid tactics)

TINY LINES: As seen in the magnifying mirror. Moisturize and lubricate skin around the clock to help stop lines from developing into wrinkles . . . avoid the sun and hot, dry air . . . stop smoking . . . drink plenty of water to keep skin plump and hydrated from within.

DRY, STIFF, ITCHY SKIN: If you insist on being a soap and water person, try rinsing twice as many times as usual, or twice as long as you currently do when you wash your face, and use cool water for rinsing. Don't dry your face, but tone with the mildest toner and apply moisturizer to damp skin . . . keep indoor air as moist as possible: spray a plant mister in the air occasionally; use an electric humidifier, a simmering tea-kettle on the stove, a water-filled tray on the radiator—anything and everything to keep humidity around you high. Slather on body lotion and hand creams, too.

DULL SKIN: Embark on a healthful eating regimen to include plenty of fresh, raw fruits and vegetables which provide essential vitamins and the fiber your body needs to clean your system; drink all the water you can to speed along the cleansing process; whip up your circulation with more vigorous exercise. If you've been sedentary, begin with twice-daily walks in the fresh air. Get more rest. Mild epidermabrasion with an abrasive cleansing puff when you clean your face will remove dead cells and help stimulate circulation near the skin surface.

INELASTIC SKIN, WHICH IS SLOW TO SPRING BACK WHEN PINCHED: Watch your diet so as to avoid losing too much weight. To be too thin is, after a certain age, far more unbecoming than gaining a few extra pounds. Provided there are no health factors involved, gaining a few pounds might make your skin appear smoother and younger. Whether you gain or maintain, be sure to keep a regular schedule of meals and rest, and to drink lots of water to keep your skin plump and hydrated.

LIVER SPOTS, OR SENILE LENTIGO: There is no known preventive measure, but for correctives you can see the dermatologist. He may advise letting the spots alone, or he may use liquid nitrogen or surgery to remove them. Often, however, the spots return in time. Some women have found the use of a bleaching cream containing 1.5 to 2 percent hydroquinone successful—but if you use this method, remember that the cream must be applied only to the spots, not to the skin around them. For spots on the face, use a concealing cover cream half a shade lighter than your foundation. To minimize spots on the hands, avoid very dark or very brilliant nail enamel or very elaborate rings and bracelets. Don't try to hide your hands, but use color and texture accents that blend with your skin rather than contrast sharply with it. For example, nail enamel in a very soft tint will flatter your hands and help minimize age spots.

BAGS AND POUCHES UNDER THE EYES: Check with your doctor to be sure a sinus or kidney problem is not involved; sleep with your head elevated on a firm pillow. Lack of exercise or rest and faulty elimination can be contributing factors as well. See the eye-makeup section for tips on minimizing bags. Remember, don't use a light concealing cover cream unless the problem is dark circles under the eyes. You can try a temporary wrinkle smoother to minimize

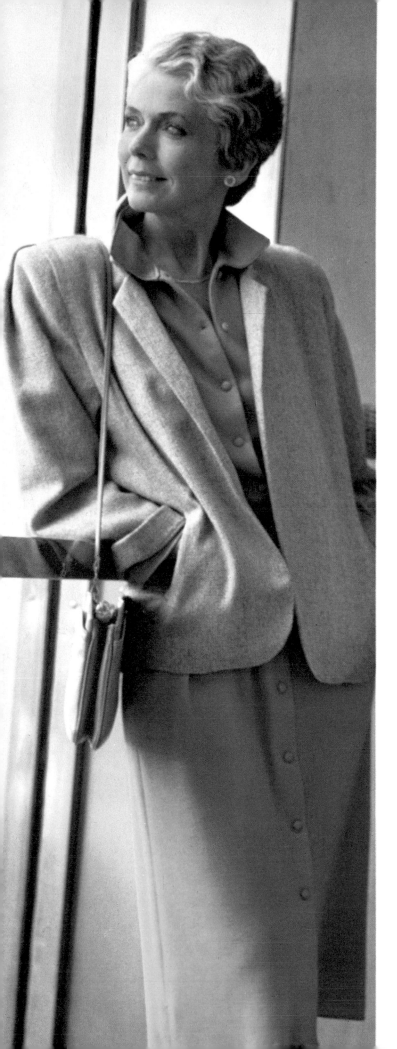

pouches. Pouchy bags will only become more apparent if light-colored cover cream is applied over them. Glasses with tinted lenses are an important fashion accessory even if your vision is 20/20. Use them to help disguise signs of aging in the eye area. Cool gray and blue-gray tints are almost universally flattering; brownish tints tend to make eyes look tired. Experiment until you discover the colors that are best for you.

DROOPING EYELIDS: Skin that overhangs the lids can be made less noticeable if you keep your eyebrows light and delicate. Be scrupulous about brow maintenance. Do not use color to darken the eyebrow, only to fill in if you must. Investigate having eyebrows lightened by a professional colorist at the hairdresser's. It is also possible to lighten the brows at home provided you use a product specially made for the purpose and are extremely careful about timing the procedure.

CROW'S FEET: Be sure to have sunglasses that are not just tinted but really dark enough to protect against glare, and be sure to wear them any time and every time you drive or go outdoors on bright days. Indoors, be sure you have adequate light for reading and other tasks. Avoid squinting, and avoid dryness—be careful to keep the skin around your eyes moisturized and lubricated at all times. Again, you can also use a temporary wrinkle smoother.

VERTICAL LINES AT THE BRIDGE OF THE NOSE: These are squinting cousins of crow's feet, produced in the same way. Prevent them from becoming more deeply etched by keeping your skin moisturized. Also wear sunglasses when outdoors, and be sure to have adequate light for indoor close-up work. Or try a temporary wrinkle smoother, which will work for a few hours. Massaging the lines at the bridge of your nose with a face cream will help to relieve tension and thus minimize lines.

WRINKLES ACROSS THE BRIDGE OF THE NOSE: Eye makeup will avoid calling attention to these lines. Use an eye shadow in a soft, light shade, and concentrate it at the outer corners of the eyes; bring shadow in no closer to the nose than the center of the eyelid. For glasses choose a frame with a deep bridge that will help camouflage the wrinkles.

WRINKLES ACROSS THE FOREHEAD: Everyone has these to some degree and often from quite a young age, so don't worry unnecessarily about these lines. You can temporarily erase them by using a wrinkle smoother. Massaging the forehead with cream will help relieve tension and thus minimize these lines as well. A hairstyle with deep bangs would hide them completely, of course, but may not be the best solution. Styles that are swept away from the face tend to give a more flattering and youthful look to the mature face. Instead of trying to hide behind hair, play up good features so as to distract the eye. Wear eye-catching earrings. Make sure your hair is as attractively styled as possible and that its color and condition are both perfect. Make your mouth and eyes the focus of your face with a color that is soft yet vibrant, and pay special attention to drawing a clear lip line. Make sure your teeth are as healthy as they look through regular visits to the dentist and scrupulous daily care. And smile often—that's the surest way to attract the eye.

VERTICAL LINES EXTENDING BEYOND THE LIPS: To avoid lipstick's "traveling" or "feathering" in these tiny lines, powder your lips before using lip color, and outline the lips with a lip pencil or brush for a lasting clear lip shape. Some lipsticks do not feather as much as others —experiment.

SAGGING CHIN AND JAWLINE: A double chin and jowls can be minimized by choice of a hairstyle with a line that curves up and out to lead the eye upward; wear flat button earrings or those with a design that follows the upward curve of the ear rather than dangling drop earrings; try wearing cowl necks, low-standing collars and loose turtlenecks, not tight high necks.

LINES IN THE SIDES OF THE CHEEKS: Wrinkling here may be a result of loss of teeth. If you are missing one or more teeth and do not wear a dental prosthesis, not only will facial wrinkles develop, but more teeth will be lost and your general health will suffer. To disguise wrinkles, use a temporary wrinkle smoother, a little concealing cover cream or a foundation a half shade lighter than your skin tone, and apply it in the hollow of the cheek. This puts to use the principle that a light color in makeup causes an area to come forward; thus the cheek will look smoother. Do not wear your hair curling onto your cheeks. Do wear light colors near your face—a collar, a scarf across the throat, earrings, a pin on the shoulder—all the attention-catching devices to focus attention away from the signs of aging skin on the cheeks.

WHEN DOES AGING START?

The individual aging pattern is unique. How you will age, and how your skin will show it, depends partly on your genes. You can get some idea of your potential pattern of lines and wrinkles by studying your parents' faces. Genes determine *where* lines will etch the skin, but when the lines will develop and how deeply is pretty much up to you. Your daily habits have a great deal to do with how your face and your body will display (or conceal!) the effects of time. Teen-agers always feel immortal and indestructible. Actually, habits formed then are often responsible for premature aging. It's never too early to form good habits . . . or too late to break bad ones. Below is a checklist of skin-saving tactics to adopt now if you want to avoid wrinkles.

DO protect your skin with moisturizer and protective sunscreens when it is exposed to sun, wind, dry heat or cold. DON'T expose your skin to any of these rough-weather conditions unnecessarily or for long periods of time if it can be avoided.

DON'T play with your face or make faces if you don't want wrinkles. Facial mannerisms—raised eyebrows, frowns, pursed lips—lead to eventual etching of the skin. Many people pick, pluck and tug idly at the skin of the face or neck, rub their eyes, or prop the chin up on an elbow or fist. These are all unconscious mannerisms and easy to develop. But they all pull at the skin, and anything that pulls at the skin works to stretch it and wrinkle it.

DO use the lightest touch when applying creams and cosmetics and always stroke upward. When applying cream around your eyes, don't stroke it on, but rather press delicately, and move from the outer corners toward the nose.

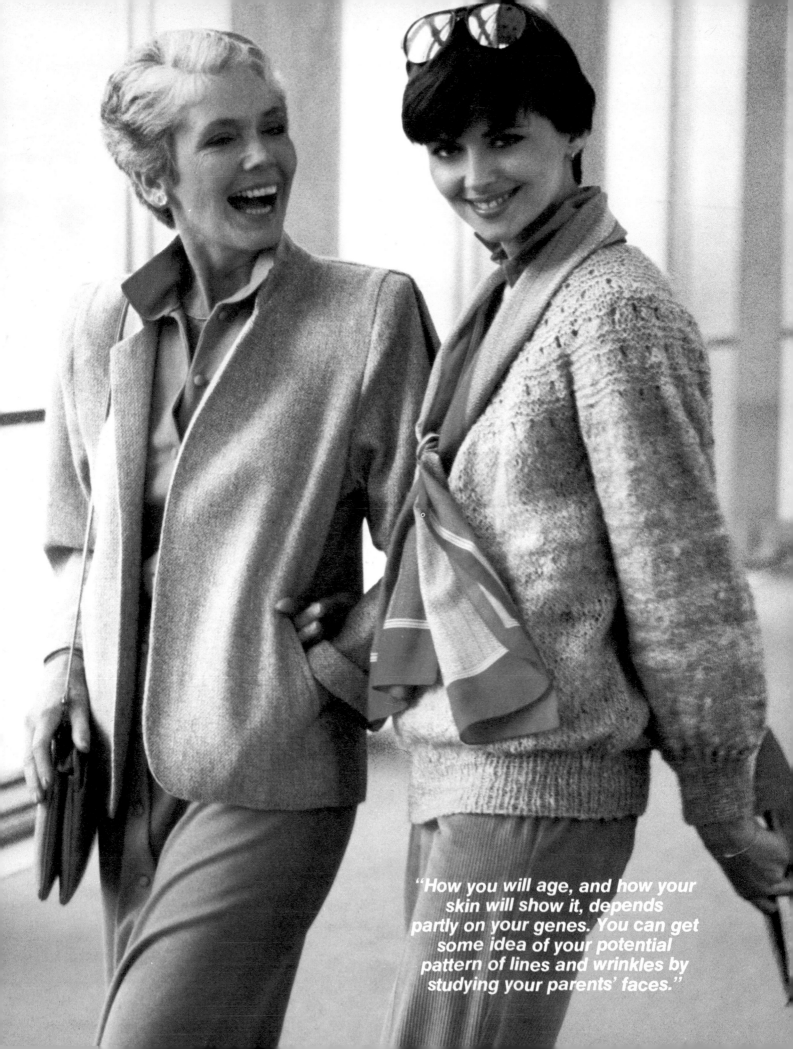

"How you will age, and how your skin will show it, depends partly on your genes. You can get some idea of your potential pattern of lines and wrinkles by studying your parents' faces."

DON'T smoke! Some dermatologists find that smokers wrinkle much more and much sooner than nonsmokers. Studies of the skins of smokers invariably show destruction of collagen —protein that holds skin together—especially around the eye area. The result is wrinkling. Breakdown of collagen around the eyes coupled with habitual squinting against the smoke leads to the familiar pattern of heavy wrinkling seen in the faces of heavy smokers.

WHY IS AGING SKIN SO DRY?

As we age, sebum-producing glands become less productive, and the cells in the underlayers of the skin retain less moisture and so lose their packing, or fullness. One of the causes is the gradual diminishing of estrogen production as we approach menopause. Therefore, a woman needs to be careful to protect her skin against external drying factors and to avoid situations that are damaging to the skin.

GETTING RID OF THE CRINKLES AND WRINKLES YOU HAVE

Prevention is easier than erasing wrinkles. Plastic surgeons dismay many prospective patients when they advise them that a face-lift cannot eliminate heavy horizontal lines on the forehead, nor can it erase vertical wrinkles above and below the lips.

For tiny vertical lines above or below the lips, dermabrasion can be employed by the plastic surgeon or a dermatologist.

For deep wrinkles on the forehead, some surgeons have had excellent results from the use of electrolysis. The electric current is used in such cases not to remove hair but to lay down a thin layer of scar tissue below the skin surface. This scar tissue raises the level of the wrinkle up to be nearly level with surrounding skin, thus minimizing the line.

Any surgery is serious, and unnecessary surgery should be avoided. Yet for a woman with the right motivation and the right expectations, cosmetic surgery may prove to be a rewarding experience. By improving her appearance, she matches the way she looks with the way she feels about herself.

Former First Lady Betty Ford, always one of the most straightforward women in the public eye, had the right motivation. "I'm sixty years old, and I wanted a nice new face to go with my beautiful new life."

Plastics surgeons try, through extensive presurgery interviews, to screen out prospective patients who have goals more ambitious than a "nice new face." A good surgeon refuses to operate on a woman who wants to regain her youth—cosmetic surgery doesn't make you look younger, just better. Similarly, he rejects the woman who wants the surgeon to transform her into a fashion magazine cover girl—surgery cannot drastically alter the structure of the face. The woman who hopes plastic surgery will "save" her marriage should be refused. Partnership between two adults is built on thousands of shared trusts and intimacies of feeling. When it goes sour, the fault lies beyond the reach of a surgeon.

The only prospective patient a reputable plastic surgeon will accept is the one the surgeon feels has no unreasonable hopes.

She (or he; an increasing number of men are seeking treatment) is someone who has a good, basically satisfying life but who wants what she considers a fault in her appearance corrected. She is a woman who wants the face and body she lives in to look as trim and alert as she feels. She views surgery not as a form of magic, but as a therapy, a technique that can be used to help her adjust better to life.

If you are seriously considering plastic surgery (and that is the only manner in which to consider it!), you should read all you can on the subject before consulting a surgeon. Several excellent books on the subject are available. You should discuss the idea with your family. Finally, if you are still convinced that surgery can be a good idea for you, ask your own physician to recommend qualified surgeons whom you might consult. Or write or call your county medical society; it can provide you with the names of surgeons who can help you. Your surgeon should have passed the exams of the American Board of Plastic Surgery. He is then said to be "board-certified." The doctor should also be a member of the American College of Surgeons, entitled to use the letters FACS (Fellow of the American College of Surgeons) after his name.

Make appointments to discuss surgery with at least two doctors. The doctors will show you before and after photographs of similar operations, and will discuss your entire medical history. They will talk with you to determine your physical and psychological preparedness for surgery. You should ask for complete information about discomfort, any possibility of scarring, and the length of recuperation.

The interview is not necessarily the prelude to surgery. Very often the surgeon or the prospective patient will decide against surgery. The surgeon may decide that the visitor is not sufficiently prepared mentally for the operation, or has unreasonable demands of surgery. A Black patient may very often be advised against surgery. The darker the skin, the more the skin tends to form keloids—thick, fibrous scar tissue. This makes surgery results on Black skin much less predictable.

Whether you are considering cosmetic surgery or not, you may want to have some idea of what is involved. Here is a brief rundown.

Face-lifts are the best-known operations in cosmetic surgery. The medical name is rhytidectomy. Facial skin is pulled up and back to soften wrinkles and eliminate sagging jowls. Sometimes muscles under the skin and jaw are tightened. Eyelid surgery is another operation. Sagging skin and fatty deposits beneath the skin are eliminated. There are also operations to augment or reduce the chin or breasts. Body lifts for arms, abdomen, buttocks, and thighs are also sometimes performed. Depending on what is done, the lasting time for the results varies from five years to a lifetime. Costs, naturally, vary considerably. But plastic surgery is not cheap. Two thousand dollars is a fairly standard outlay for eyelid surgery.

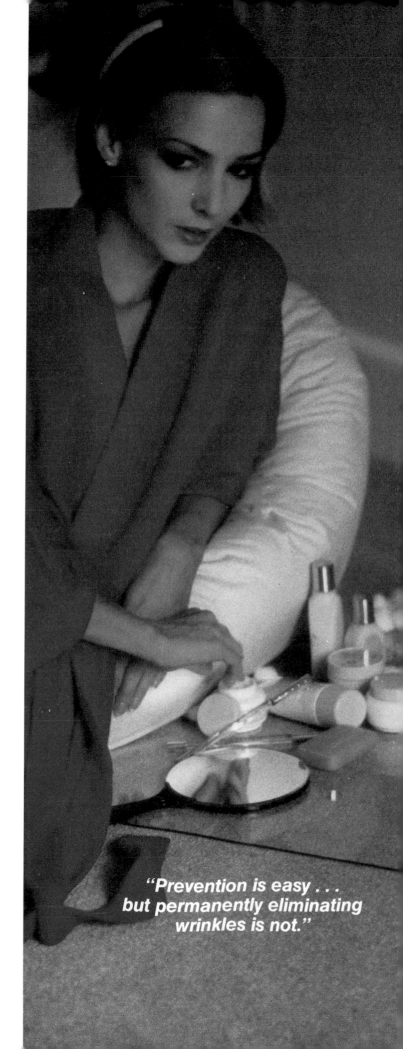

"Prevention is easy . . . but permanently eliminating wrinkles is not."

Some time in the sun

You know how to make raisins, don't you? Take some plump, juicy grapes with smooth, satiny skin and put them in the sun for a while. Have you looked at a raisin lately? What the sun does for grapes, it can also do to your skin.

Prevention is easy, but permanently eliminating wrinkles is not.

This does not mean you need to live like a mole, shunning ski trips and days at the beach, but you cannot play fast-and-loose with the sun. Sun damage—solar aging, the dermatologists call it—is cumulative and irreversible. Every year hundreds of thousands of Americans are treated for skin cancers, and most of those cancers are directly traceable to sun exposure. It is not one bad sunburn that does the damage, but a steady buildup of time in the sun over the years, time in which ultraviolet rays gradually break down collagen and elastin in the skin. Tanning is a pigment change undergone by the skin in order to protect itself from the danger of excessive ultraviolet rays.

Not total spoilsports, dermatologists say that *some* sun is all right, and may even be beneficial. A little sun exposure is needed for the body to synthesize vitamin D. However, it takes only nineteen square inches of skin and five minutes of sun a day to provide all the vitamin D you need. Some dermatologists will even admit that people feel healthier and more attractive with a slight rosy golden glow from the sun. The important thing to remember is that whenever you are exposed to the sun for any length of time, you should protect your skin with a sunscreen. That's imperative!

Although every skin is affected by the sun, not every skin reacts to sun exposure in the same way. People whose ancestors were from northern climates fare worst in the sun. Those with blue eyes, particularly if their forebears were Celtic (Welsh, Scots, Irish) may have the worst time. Often, they get pink or ruddy but never tan—they burn, and even worse, they blister; they are more likely to develop cancers from sun exposure. Olive-skinned people, and those whose ancestors came from the Mediterranean basin, generally fare better in the sun. Black skins can burn, freckle or tan, depending on the individual. All skins generally have the same number of melanocytes (the cells that produce the tanning pigment melanin), but not all melanocytes are equally productive. And the efficiency of the melanin production varies with age. Children can tolerate only about half as much sun as adults, and infants and toddlers can take far less than older children. Later in life, sun tolerance may decline sharply. So just because you haven't burned so far, don't think you are immune.

Solar radiation varies in intensity depending on where you are and when. It is at its maximum on June 21 at the equator. The atmosphere affords some protection from the sun. At the seashore, where the atmosphere is densest, you have more sun protection than in the mountains, where the atmosphere is thinner. The danger in the mountains is especially great in winter, because of snow glare. A sunburn can develop in less than fifteen minutes in the tropics; the farther north of the equator, the longer you are likely to be able to remain in the sun without burning. And you are apt to be safer on Labor Day than earlier in the summer, not only because radiation is less intense, but because you are more likely to have built up some tan protection.

Not all tanning products contain sunscreens, but *only* sunscreens will allow you to tan while giving you protection against burning. Several different chemicals are effective when used in sunscreens. The best is generally agreed to be PABA (para-aminobenzoic acid) and its derivatives. Other effective sunscreen agents are cinnamates, or cinoxate, homosalates, and benzophenones (there are several, all with the suffix "-benzone," which you'll find on the label).

In August, 1978, the Food and Drug Administration proposed a system of numbers to rate the Sun Protection Factor of a sunscreen. The higher the SPF number, the greater the degree of protection the product affords the user.

To take advantage of the FDA recommendations, choose according to your skin. Here's how it works. SPF numbers are Factor 2 (minimal protection), Factor 4 (moderate), Factor 6 (extra) and Factor 8 (maximum protection). There is also a lone odd number. That's Factor 15, and it is used for a virtual sun block which does not allow tanning at all.

It isn't necessary to stay with the same Factor number all summer: you can start with a Factor 8; then, once you acquire a base tan, move on to Factor 4. Once you have got as dark as you wish, however, you can begin using a higher Factor again, to avoid getting too dark. And you can use products with different Factor numbers at the same time on different parts of your body. Very vulnerable, thin-skinned areas should always be more protected. It's wise to use a higher-Factor product on nose, eye area, throat and V of the chest and backs of the hands and knees, even when you use a lower Factor for protecting the rest of the body, where skin is thicker.

Timing, even with a sunscreen, is important. You should apply your sunscreen carefully and thoroughly thirty minutes before going into the sun. And remember to reapply it. Water robs skin of sunscreen protection; so does perspiration. Even when sitting under a beach umbrella, or in dappled shade, reapply sunscreen after two hours; if perspiring, within thirty minutes and right after a swim.

In addition to sunscreens, there are *sun blocks*. These reflect ultraviolet light rays off the skin and prevent both burning and tanning. Most are opaque. Zinc oxide, the white paste lifeguards often wear on nose and lips, is the most common. If you are allergic to the sun, you should use a sun block.

"Tanning lotions" and "tanning oils" without sunscreen ingredients afford no protection for the skin, other than lubricating it. Coconut oil, baby oil with iodine, and so on, just smell nice and lubricate. They don't protect.

The so-called "instant tanning" products contain dihydroxyacetone (DHA), which colors the skin. They are generally judged safe to use, but they afford no protection against burning.

If you are really protective of your skin, you'll watch the clock no matter how carefully you have applied sunscreen. Maximum first exposure should be no more than fifteen minutes.

" . . . don't just lie there in the sun"

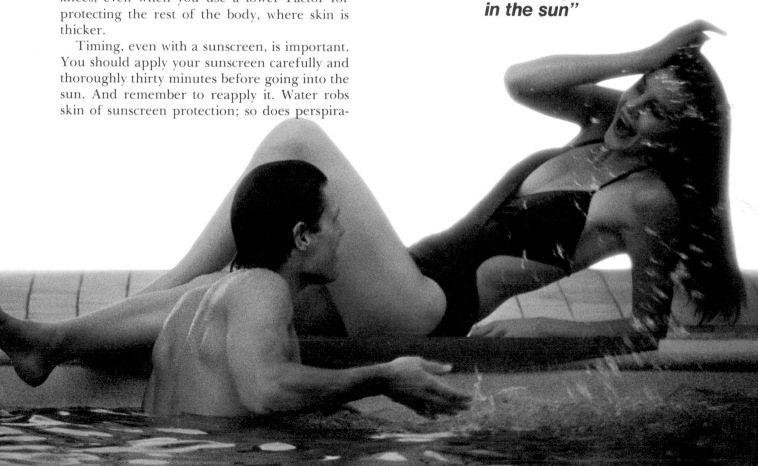

Add five minutes next day, five minutes more the next. Never take the sun when it's at its zenith, if you can avoid it. Just ten minutes in the sun at noon can do more damage than thirty minutes before 11 A.M. or after 3 P.M. From 12 to 2, "Even caribou lie around and snooze" in Noël Coward's song, while "mad dogs and Englishmen go out in the mid-day sun." If, like the misguided colonials in the song, you "detest a siesta," you'd be smart to go in for lunch or some other undercover activity at noon.

Sun Protection Factor Chart		
Skin Type	*SPF*	*Protection*
A. Always burns easily, never tans, sensitive	8 to 15	Maximum to Ultra
B. Always burns easily, tans minimally, sensitive	6 to 8	Maximum
C. Usually burns slightly, tans gradually	4 to 6	Moderate
D. Seldom burns, tans easily	2 to 4	Minimal
E. Rarely burns, gets very dark tan	2	Minimal

■ Remember you need added protection for delicate skin around the eyes, on the throat and on the backs of the hands, and apply extra sunscreen.

TIPS IN THE SUN

DON'T

■ Don't use a sun reflector or a metallic reflector blanket. Serious burns, even fatalities, have resulted from their use.

■ Don't be fooled by haze or clouds. Maximum cloud cover blocks only about half the burning rays; haze can reflect, and you burn badly.

■ Don't think you are safe under a beach umbrella. Rays reflected off sand and water can burn you from the sides, and most umbrellas block only about half the rays that come from directly above.

DO

■ Wear good dark sunglasses any time you are in the sun, winter or summer. Be sure they are dark enough to allow only 20 to 30 percent light transmission if you are serious about protecting your eyes. If your eyes can be seen easily through the glasses, the glasses aren't dark enough.

■ Remember that medications (antibiotics, diuretics, antihistamines, tranquilizers, oral contraceptives and sugar substitutes, for example) can cause skin to have a photosensitive reaction—irritation or a quick, bad sunburn.

AFTER THE SUN

The nicest way to follow a time in the sun is with a quick, refreshing, tepid shower. It's a delicious way to pamper your skin and your psyche. Wash away the heat of day; then pat yourself dry very gently. Soothe your damp skin all over with your favorite after-shower fragrance treat. It makes your skin feel cool and wonderful, and helps your tan look better and last longer.

SOOTHE YOUR SKIN

If you have miscalculated your exposure time or used the wrong Factor number and discover you are severely burned, see a doctor.

Sunburn-pain-reliever sprays are effective in less severe cases. As an alternative, if you have it handy, pour two cups of oatmeal flakes into a piece of cheesecloth, tie it into a bag and toss into the bathtub. Draw a bath that's slightly cooler than body temperature. (Test as you would a baby's formula: try a little of the water on your wrist. It should feel faintly cool on the skin.) As you soak—allow ten minutes or so—the oatmeal solution helps soothe the skin.

If eyes are sunburned and swollen, soothe them with compresses made from fresh cucumber slices or a cold-water compress. This works to help reduce swelling.

Another effective pain reliever for sunburn is a wet handkerchief saturated with a solution of vinegar and water (about 50–50 is the most comfortable proportion).

WHAT ABOUT VITAMINS?

Of course vitamins can help your skin—they help every part of you—but just as you don't sing one note of a song, you don't take only one vitamin for your skin. Vitamins work in concert, each one dependent on the others. Through your diet, and in supplements, you should aim for at least the U.S. Government's RDA (Rec-ommended Daily Allowance) of all the essential vitamins and minerals.

Some people believe that if vitamins can help skin from inside out, they can work in reverse, too, and they advocate using vitamins directly on the skin. The idea is that a capsule of vitamin A or vitamin E, pricked open with a needle, can be smeared directly on the skin, where it will promote healing of blemishes, scars, burns or wounds. Most dermatologists, however, question their effectiveness.

"Walk, run, play tennis, sail, ski, but do something to keep moving so that you even out the exposure."

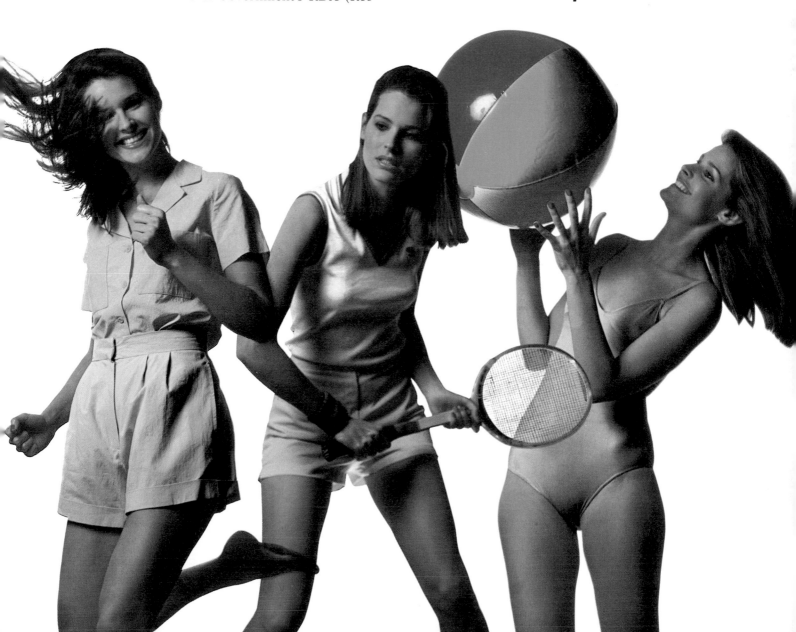

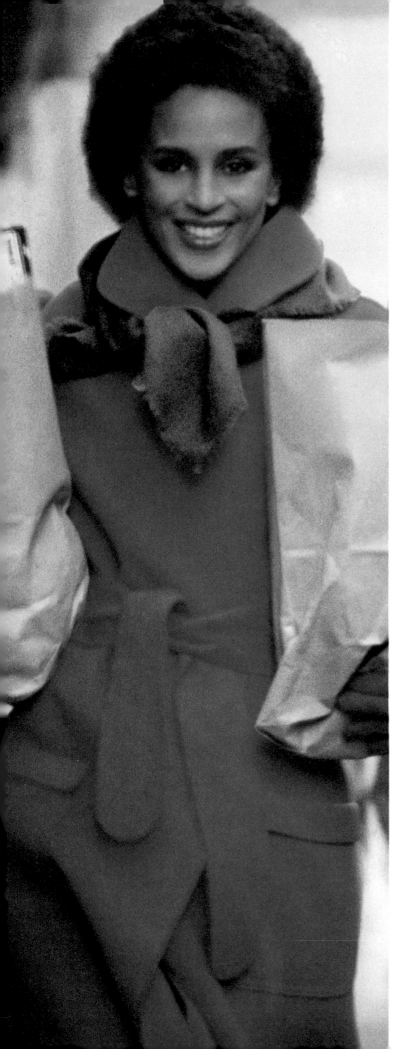

SKIN CARE BY THE SEASONS

Skin care changes with the seasons. Cold, dry air and hot, dry air are equally bad for skin. Very bad. And we have to contend with both kinds in the course of a winter day. We go from cold, dry air outdoors into steam heat that's dry as the Sahara.

BEFORE GOING OUT IN THE COLD

Winterize your skin. You'd do as much for your car, wouldn't you?

Moisturize well; protect your eyes with eye cream or an extra dab of moisturizer on the delicate skin around the eyes. You want a somewhat glowing face in cold weather, a less matte finish to makeup on winter days. Cream blush and cream eye shadows are a great idea in cold, dry weather, when even oily skin tends to be slow about producing natural moisture. Lips need lots of protection against chapping in the cold, so creamy lipstick and gloss are essential. Be lavish with moisture lotion for your body. Dry skin is a real hazard in winter, especially on hands and legs. Don't neglect pedicures in winter to keep feet comfortable and smooth inside boots. Treat your feet to cream after the bath, and follow with powder to keep them comfortable and dry (important since boots trap perspiration inside, and that's bad for the skin). Use a hand cream, and don't forget cuticle cream around your nails—it won't harm your manicure, and definitely will help your hands. Gloves have made a definite fashion comeback. It makes good sense to protect hands with gloves in cold weather, and good fashion sense, too. For your hair, regular conditioning is a must during the cold weather. Hair, like skin, tends to dry in freezing temperatures and can actually break. Keep your head covered when outside: a warm head keeps you warm all over. But take your hat off indoors. A hat or cap worn in overheated stores while shopping, in the office or at home will cause perspiration to be trapped on the scalp and in the hair, which ruins your hairstyle.

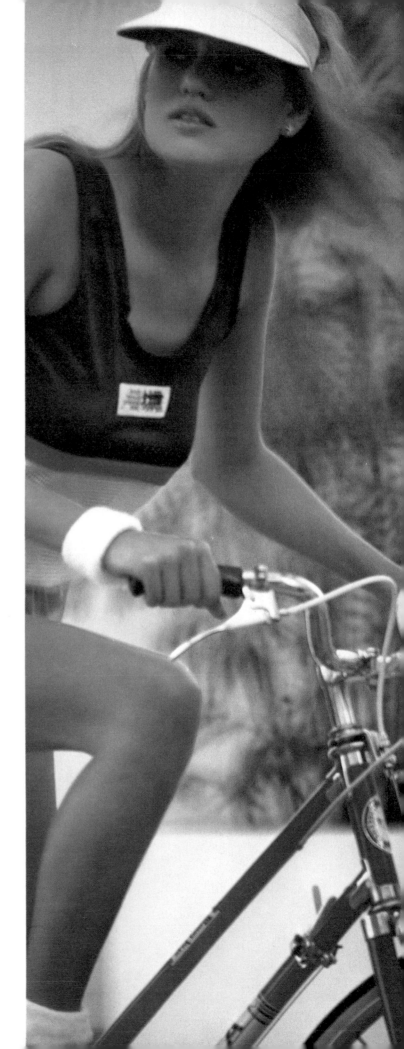

SUMMERPROOF YOUR SKIN

Warm weather makes us feel more relaxed and active, invigorates our skin. Cell production and turnover is more rapid, oil glands more active. All that, plus a little sunshine and fresh air, adds up to better-looking skin for almost everyone. Although many minor skin annoyances seem to clear up spontaneously and disappear, you do have to keep up skin care every day. Skin care and makeup products containing suncreen are especially important at this time of year. Moisturizer is important on those days when you use next-to-no makeup. It protects your skin and also helps make your complexion look more even and glowing. Use moisturizer or eye cream around your eyes, especially. Lubrication helps prevent crinkle lines you get from squinting against bright daylight and glare. What helps even more is to lubricate the skin around the eyes, then protect the eyes with dark glasses so you don't have to squint.

You can lose body heat through your extremities in hot weather as well as cold. To cool your whole body quickly, rinse feet and wrists in cold water, or stroke an ice cube on wrists. Follow up with a splash or a spray of cologne.

Makeup is lighter in summer, and you will look better with just the right touches. Eyes get "lost" in a tan unless you give them importance and definition. Mascara and delicate eyeliner are very important. When it's humid, try using either waterproof makeup or powder shadows and blush colors; you may find they're neater than creams for hot, steamy days. Lipstick and gloss are essentials for a pretty summer face. All the ripe colors of summer fruits are delectable —watermelon, plum, cherry, raspberry, peach and apricot look as good as they sound. Summer roses should bloom on the cheeks, but contouring looks heavy and wintry. Just plant a blush high on the apples of your cheeks, and maybe a little color above the bridge of your nose and across the forehead, where the sun would strike. You'll look healthy and terrific.

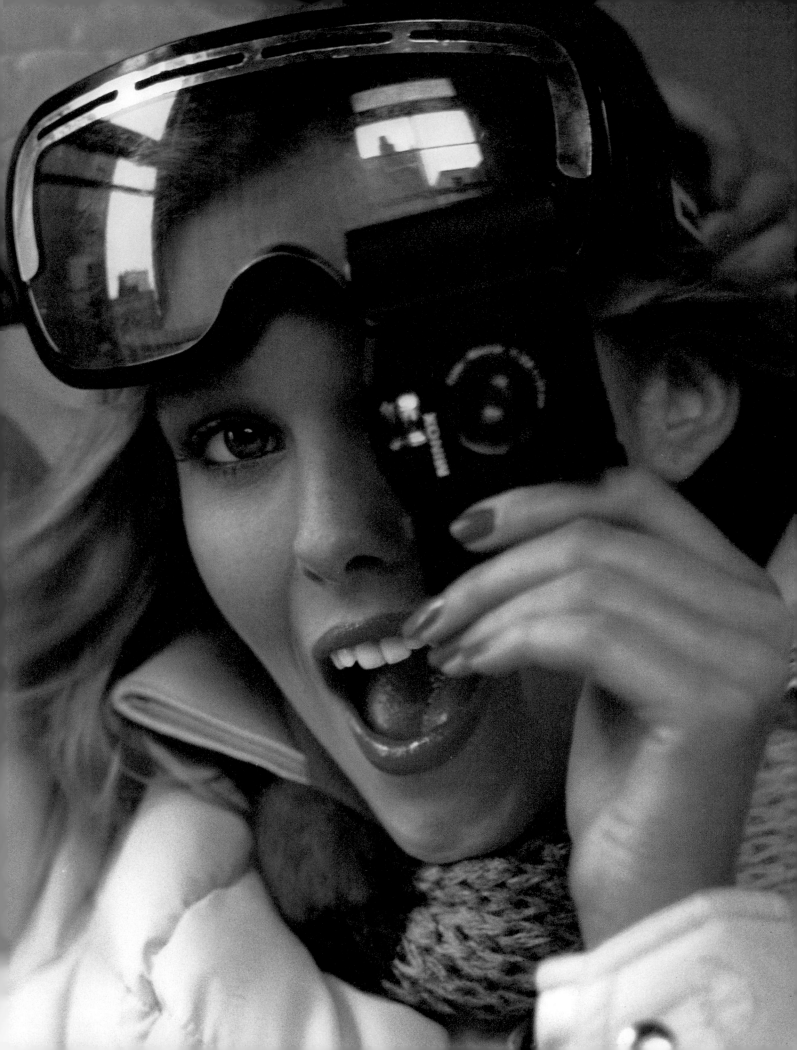

WHEN YOU TURN WINTER INTO SUMMER, AND VICE VERSA

Some women are lucky enough to be able to escape when the icy winds and snows start, but when you trade climates quickly, remember it takes your skin a while to adjust. Skin adapts slowly to climate changes. Cell turnover and sebum production speed up gradually in summer, slow down gradually in winter. When you take a jet from snow to sandy beach, skin is unprepared and needs help in adjusting.

WHEN YOU GO FROM COLD TO WARM WEATHER

■ Be extra careful about the sun. In the tropics, sun is more dangerous than at home. You're closer to the equator, so the sun is nearer. Also, it's probably been several months, at least, since your last exposure to sun. Use the right sunscreen, and limit first-day exposure to fifteen minutes at a time, for a total of no more than forty-five minutes to an hour. If you use a sunscreen with a very high Factor right at the start, you will enjoy your vacation in the sun, not indoors with a sunburn.
■ Moisturize all over and frequently. Add oil to the water if you bathe.

WHEN YOU GO FROM WARM TO COLD WEATHER

■ Protect your skin from cold, dry weather. Moisturize; use lip gloss, hand cream. Use a sunscreen, too, if you go out in the snow. Sun is fierce at high altitudes, and so is snow glare.
■ Protect your eyes with eye cream and goggles or dark glasses from wind, sun and cold. Have a warm bath after coming home from the cold, use bath oil in the water and lots of body cream when you get out of the tub.

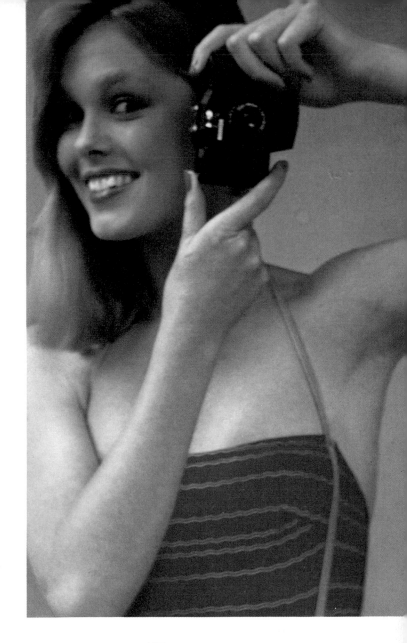

"Be sure to use a good sunscreen and limit first day exposure to the sun."

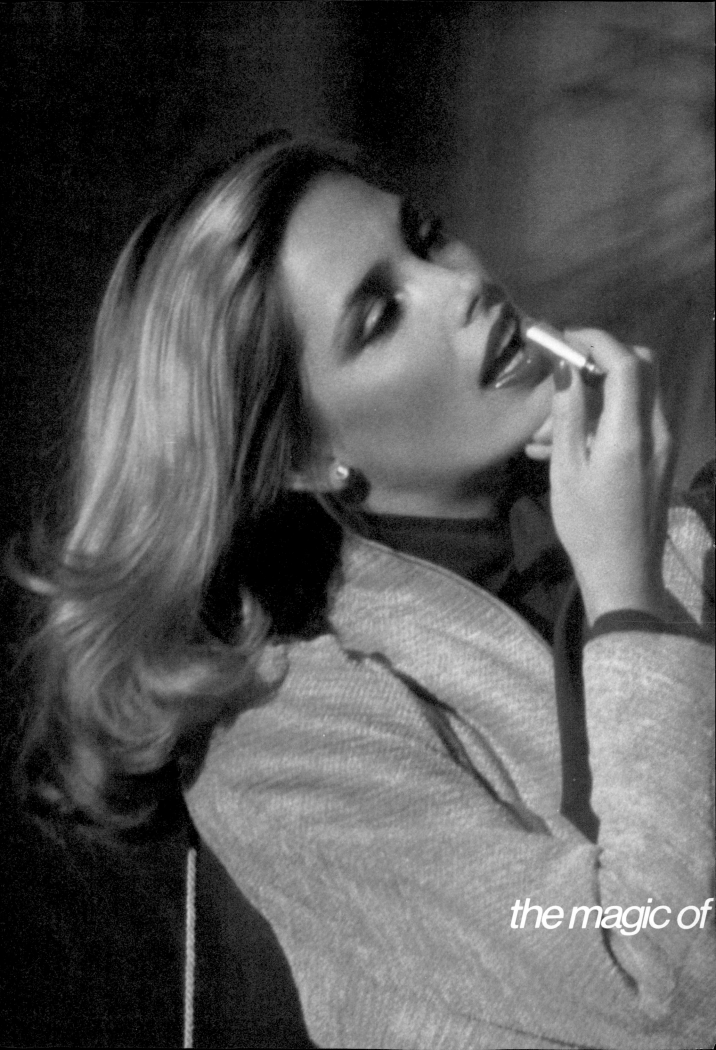

the magic of

MAKEUP

Play with makeup

Makeup can create magic effects, either subtle or dramatic, but for some women makeup suggests heavy application and complicated directions. But in reality, it is surprisingly easy, and fun, to become an artist with makeup. If you practice the art, you can learn how to bring your own best features to the fore, to make your face come alive *without* ever looking "made up." Models and actresses aren't born knowing how to apply makeup. They learn, as everyone must, and they keep practicing and changing. A model spends her off hours trying out new makeup tricks just for fun, perfecting her skills. She doesn't wait until just before the camera starts clicking.

It's a model's stock in trade, of course, but every woman should become familiar with the texture and contours of her face and then devote a few minutes of her time every now and then to perfecting her makeup skills. Try a new way with eye makeup some rainy afternoon, or during your Beauty Time this week. Then when a big evening comes along, it will be a simple matter to do your eyes in a glamorous new way. Through practice you become familiar and comfortable with the tools and techniques that can help you look your best.

Even more important, practice helps you become familiar with your own face. Does that sound odd? You've spent a lifetime looking at your face, but how much time have you spent in feeling the bones under the skin? To bring out your cheekbones with makeup, to know where to apply your blush, you must know right where the bones are, and you can know that only by exploring your face with your fingers. What you need now is self-knowledge.

After you have taken your luxurious beauty bath, study the texture of your facial skin. Is the texture fine or coarse; is the condition dry or oily? Use your fingers to explore the texture of your skin and to feel around for the underlying bone structure. Sit before the mirror in natural daylight if at all possible, so that you get the truest picture of the state of your skin, hair and eye color today. If the evening is your special Beauty Time, be sure you have a good quantity of white light to help you in your self-assessment. Don't use fluorescent lighting, because it tends to dull and wash out red tones while emphasizing blues.

Now you are ready to make a list of your goals with makeup. Decide which are your best features and how you can learn to play them up. You don't want to concentrate on eye makeup to the exclusion of everything else—that sort of unbalanced face is completely outdated—but you will want to practice all the little enhancements for pretty eyes, as well as discover which lipstick colors can create a well-shaped, sensuous mouth; how to use different colors for a glowing blush; how to choose a foundation to enhance your skin.

Talking about makeup can make it seem complicated. It's not. You'll be surprised at how quick and easy these methods and tips really are. If it *looks* time-consuming, that's because every little step is explained in the directions. That's to make it easy to do, whether you're skilled or taking your first flyer with makeup. It's the opposite of those recipes sometimes passed along by very experienced cooks that say, "Bake until it's done." Sounds simple until you realize that you have no idea how high the oven temperature should be, or how it looks when it is done.

"Use your fingers to explore your underlying bone structure."

GETTING ORGANIZED

Your choice of makeup colors and products is almost as individual as a fingerprint. As you read this chapter, you might enjoy making a list of new things you'd like to try—new little treats you can add to the makeup you're now using, or products that will help you make some attractive changes in your makeup plans. There are some basic products and little tools that every home makeup tray should include in order to be complete. Below are suggestions for a makeup collection at home, as well as for a carry-along kit.

AT HOME:

Cleanser

Moisturizer/Toner

Foundation (to match skin tone)

Concealer (½ shade lighter than skin tone)

Blusher

Pressed powder

Loose powder

Lip pencils, lipstick and lip gloss

Eye shadow (more than one color)

Tissues

Sterile cotton balls or pads

Cotton swabs

Tweezers

Eyelash curler

Eyebrow brush

Powder brush

Mascara

Eyeliner

Eyebrow pencil

AWAY FROM HOME: This kit is planned to be kept at work, if you have facilities there to keep personal belongings. It's also a good idea to have a makeup kit for travel all stocked and ready for an overnight trip. The key to this kit is size—*small* bottles, *small* sizes of everything. There's no need for a whole box of cotton swabs, only a couple; and, of course, loose powder stays at home. Otherwise, your carry-along kit can have everything you normally use at home, yet fit neatly into a waterproof (that's important!) plastic bag hardly bigger than your hand.

AND DON'T FORGET . . .

When you're going out for a short time or for the day, you should have a little bare-bones mini kit in your purse. Include only those things which need to be refreshed: lip color, blush, pressed powder, purse fragrance spray.

THE STEPS TO A PERFECT, FINISHED MAKEUP

Every woman works out her own favorite pattern of doing things, whether it's making a bed or making up. But since we're on the subject of trying out new ideas and fresh new ways of doing things, you might enjoy reviewing your sequence of applying makeup and checking it against the one most professional makeup artists advise:

1. Brow shaping and maintenance (Note—it is preferable to tweeze brows at night and apply makeup next morning so that skin is recovered from any irritation).

2. Cleansing, toning, moisturizing—the imperative first steps that precede any makeup.

3. Concealing cover cream—This step is optional, and you may not need it.

4. Foundation—See pages 52–53.

5. Contour and shading—another optional step, primarily for evening.

6. Powder—depending on the form of eye and cheek colors you use. See page 56.

7. Blusher—See pages 57–59.

8. Eye shadow—See pages 61–63.

9. Eyeliner—See pages 64–65.

10. Eyelash curling—See page 65.

11. Mascara—See page 65.

12. Brow coloring—if necessary; often it is not. See page 50.

13. Powder—If not used before, powder is the finishing step. See page 55.

14. Lipstick and gloss—see pages 67–69.

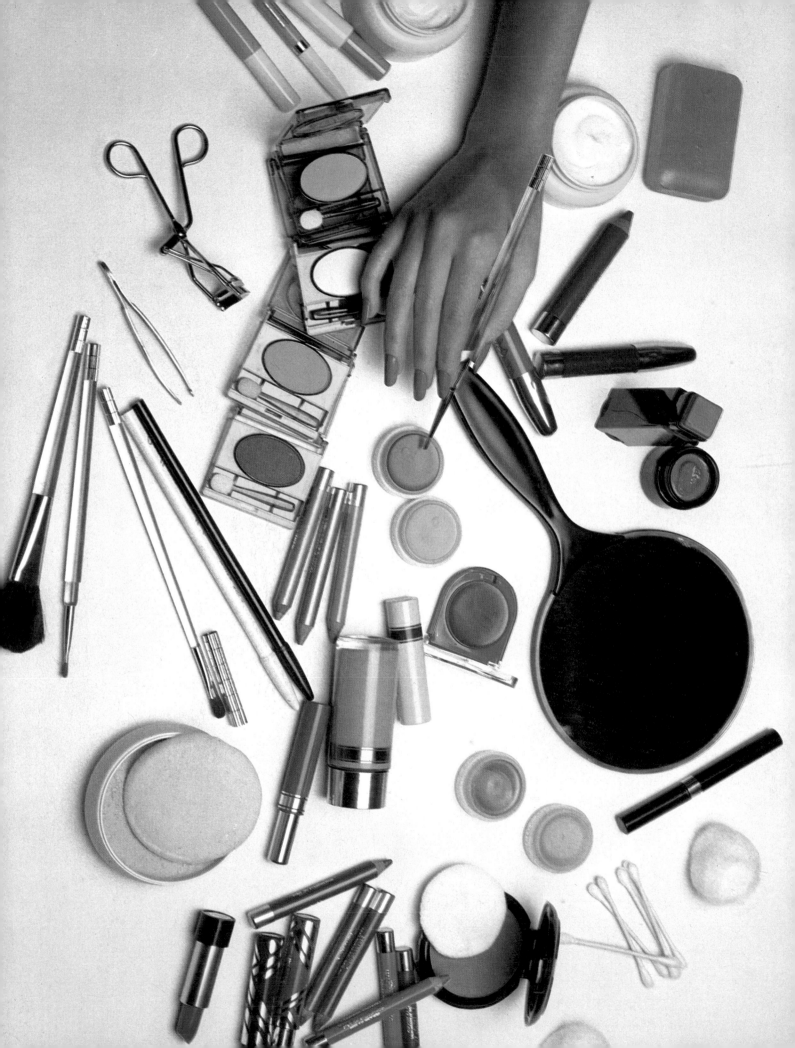

THE NATURAL BROW

Your eyebrows define the mood of your entire face and provide a mobile frame for your eyes. Let the drama come from your eyes—keep eyebrows natural, in proportion to the size of your eyes, and neat. Pencil-thin brows à la Dietrich, aggressive brows like Joan Crawford's—eyebrow drama of that sort belongs on *The Late Show,* not on your face for the 1980s.

The natural brow is not only the most flattering for your face, it's also the easiest to have. These sketches show you how to use a pencil and a mirror to find where your eyebrows should begin, arch and end.

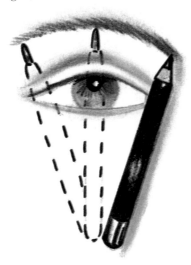

Maintenance is a simple matter, but there is a right time for it and a proper procedure. The right time is at night, after cleansing and toning but before moisturizing or applying night cream. This allows any redness or irritation of the skin that tweezing might produce to subside overnight before you make up in the morning. Saturate a cotton ball with alcohol or skin toner and use the wet pad to remove any trace of oil from brows or fingers. Cleanse tweezers with alcohol. Make sure you have a good light and preferably a magnifying mirror. Hold skin taut between thumb and forefinger. Pluck in the direction of hair growth, one hair at a time. Tweeze any unwanted hair from below the brow and between the brows, but do not tweeze above

the brow. Finish by wiping the brow with a cotton pad dampened with skin toner.

Most professional makeup artists advise that you leave eyebrow pencil as the last step of your makeup. The reasoning is that the makeup can be thrown off balance if the eyebrows are too dark and that overdarkening the brow is all too easy to do. A very dark eyebrow can give the face a hard or threatening look, and make eyes seem smaller.

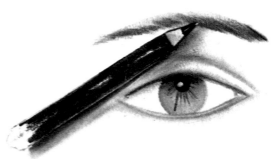

After making up your eyes as described on pages 61–65, you may find that you need only brush your eyebrows for a finished and balanced look. There are specially designed brushes that are ideal for brushing brows upward then out into a smooth, natural arch.

If you need color to define the shape of your eyebrows or to fill in sparse areas, here are some pointers: Most brows need little or no darkening; if you use a pencil, go slowly, and stop to check as you go along. The eyebrow should not be one hard, sharp pencil line but made up of delicate, feathery strokes like little individual

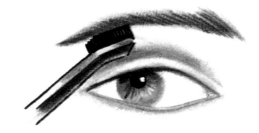

hairs. Keep your pencil very sharp, and draw in these little hairlike strokes in the direction of growth. If you accidentally darken the brow too heavily, remove some of the color with a brush or a cotton swab.

UNDERCOVER WORK

A creamy concealer can be a fabulous tool for lightening circles under your eyes or camouflaging dark marks on your skin. There are some basic tricks to using it, however. Here they are:

DO use concealer stick after moisturizing and before foundation.

DON'T go too light. Choose a concealer shade that is a half shade lighter than your own skin tone. A very light concealer will call attention to itself, even under foundation.

DO apply concealer *just below,* rather than directly on, the dark undereye circles, and blend up into the dark area. Dot on, starting at the corner of the eye, continuing toward the hairline. Then blend with a featherlight touch.

DON'T try to lighten the area drastically. Slight shadowing under the eye looks more natural.

DON'T use a concealer if the problem is not dark circles but rather puffiness. A light concealer will cause bags to come forward visually and so look worse. A temporary wrinkle smoother will minimize the bags. Sleeping with your head slightly raised helps prevent undereye puffiness. And remember, fresh cucumber slices or cotton balls soaked with witch hazel really work wonders on puffy eyes.

DO dot concealer directly on blemishes and blend with fingertips.

DO use two light applications of concealer rather than one heavy application.

Three women—one in her 20's, one in her 30's, one in her 40's . . .

Your own technique makes makeup work wonders. Watch how. Here, and on the following pages, three women follow three very individual makeup plans. In each case, the plan is the one best suited to her age, her skin and bone structure. The product form each uses—cream, powder, stick—is as always a purely personal matter of choice. Here are three different directions to beauty, first getting underway with undercover work.

In her twenties (top), this woman dots blemishes with concealer to blend with a fingertip. In her thirties (center), this woman blends out patches of uneven color through sparing use of a concealer stick that almost exactly matches her skin. In her forties (bottom), this woman uses concealer lightly just below (not on) dark undereye circles.

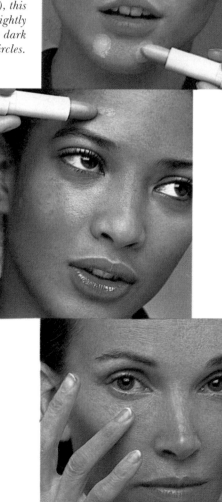

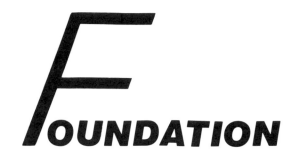

FOUNDATION

GRAND ILLUSION

The beautiful illusion of flawless skin is what foundation offers. Properly chosen and applied, foundation smooths and evens the tone and texture of the skin, causing little imperfections to become less apparent. It provides a velvet-smooth base over which eye and cheek colors glide on easily; unlike the old unnatural-looking pancake makeup that clogged pores, today's foundations are formulated to help the skin look natural and often contain sunscreen and other protective ingredients.

You might not choose to wear foundation every day, and if your skin is very good, you might not choose to wear foundation all over. But the right foundation is an indispensable aid to a really beautiful, subtle makeup.

There are two basic kinds of foundation: Liquid and Cream. Each is available in three formulations:

OIL-BASED—As the name implies, the color is suspended in oil. You must be very skillful in order to avoid a heavy look when working with oil-based foundation.

WATER-BASED—Only a tiny amount of oil, emulsified with lots of water, acts as the medium of suspension that holds the color. A water-based foundation goes on smoothly and easily for a natural look, and also helps moisturize the skin. This is the most popular kind and is excellent for normal to dry skin.

OIL-FREE—The color is held in a medium that contains no animal, mineral or vegetable oils, and some even absorb oils from the skin. Best for oily and troubled-oily skin.

Next, select the best finish for you. There are three finishes:

DEWY gives a moist, glowing look to normal or dry skin. A dewy finish helps minimize tiny lines on mature skin.

MATTE gives a smooth, even, no-shine look on normal or oily skin.

SEMI-MATTE gives a smooth, even effect suitable for all skin types.

Choose the degree of coverage you want. This ranges from almost transparent *Sheer,* which evens out color on near-perfect complexions, through *Light* and *Medium,* which help conceal flaws, to *Ultra* or *Heavy* coverage, which can alter skin tone and help conceal blemishes.

Finally, there is the question of shade. The right shade will blend to invisibility on your skin. And that is done by matching your skin tone as closely as you possibly can. Take the time to get this right. Remember, the effect of the finished makeup depends on the foundation.

1. Choose foundation in natural daylight. Your skin and foundation tones can be matched most easily in the truest light.
2. You will be wearing foundation on your face, so that's the place to try it. Yes, you *could* try it on the back of your hand, but why take half measures with such an important choice as your foundation? Besides, many makeup artists argue that skin on the face is subtly (but definitely) different in tone from skin on the rest of the body. You can prove it by holding the back of your hand up next to your cheek (before applying makeup, of course) and looking in the mirror.
3. Blend a dot of foundation into clean skin along the jaw or on the forehead. Let it set for a couple of seconds, then check. If the foundation shows up as a patch of ivory, peach or any other color against the rest of your skin, pass it by. But if you can't find where the foundation ends, if it blends invisibly into your natural skin tone, you've found the right shade.

THE BEST WAY TO APPLY FOUNDATION

Apply foundation after cleansing, toning, moisturizing and, if it's part of your makeup plan, after using a concealer.

Apply lightly and sparingly with a clean fingertip across cheeks, along nose, across forehead, across eyelids and along chin.

Blend up and out over the skin wherever foundation is needed to smooth and even out skin tone. If you have good skin, you needn't cover your face entirely. Do cover tiny discolorations, broken capillaries, veins in the eyelids and shiny patches. If you use foundation over areas where there is downy fuzz, such as the upper lip, use it sparingly because foundation will accentuate the hair.

Be careful to avoid getting foundation into the hairline, as the effect is very unattractive. To help prevent this, use a ribbon or towel to hold your hair off your face.

Feather out the foundation with smooth upward and outward strokes. Then blend down along the jawbone and feather out along the underside of the jawbone. There should be no line of demarcation where the foundation stops (that's why choosing the shade closest to your natural skin tone is so important), and blending makeup down the neck leads to unsightly collar rings.

KEEP YOUR FOUNDATION SHADE CURRENT

Even for those women who don't actively seek a suntan there is bound to be some exposure to the sun, and most often that's enough to cause your skin to be slightly darker in summer, slightly paler in winter. As you would change your wardrobe for summer, change your foundation. Select a sheer coverage formula in a slightly darker shade than your winter foundation. To make a gradual, natural transition from lighter to darker, use the palm of your hand to mix a drop of the new, darker foundation with your current one. Gradually increase the proportion of dark to light over the tanning season, then reverse as your tan fades in the fall.

3 IMPORTANT TIPS
ON FOUNDATION

1. When you apply foundation, start with the smallest amount you think possible. Blending a small amount is easier than working with too much foundation. It's easier, too, to apply a little more foundation if you need it than it is to remove an excess without streaking.

2. Use your lightest touch when blending foundation around the eye area (your ring finger or little finger is weakest, therefore best to use for applying and blending makeup near the eyes). Skin around the eyes is delicate and susceptible to pulling. Skin here also contains tiny lines in which surplus makeup will tend to cake.

3. Very good skins and very dark skins always look best with a very sheer foundation.

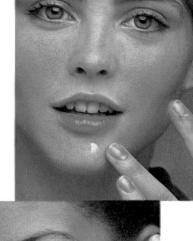

For a young woman with oily skin, top, oil-free foundation is the answer. Center, normal-to-dry skin gets smooth-flowing color with a moisturizing foundation. Below, mature skin, which tends to be drier, welcomes a soft, dewy finish and medium coverage to minimize tiny lines.

SPECIAL EFFECTS: SHADE AND CONTOUR

In the movie business, an Academy Award is given for Special Effects. Makeup artists deserve some kind of award for the special effects they can achieve with powders and creams to shade and contour a face. A clever makeup artist can create a slim, symmetrical face with perfect features no matter what the bare face looks like. To the camera, at least, the shading and contouring will be undetectable.

The makeup artist works on the idea that light reveals, dark conceals. To bring out a feature, use a light color on it. To minimize it, a dark one.

That's the theory. And it works. But it works best in pictures. In real life, changing the shape of a face with light, shadow and color is a tricky bit of business. When your artistry is too noticeable it seems to work in reverse. Say, for example, you want to narrow a round face. In principle, you would use a dark matte color in a triangle just below the cheekbones. This is to make the cheekbones seem higher and make the cheeks look less plump. In practice, it usually looks as though there is some kind of dark smudge on your round cheeks. Since that's so unusual, eyes tend to focus right on the area you would prefer to have ignored.

It is much better, as a rule, to use makeup skill constructively. Spend time on really terrific eye makeup. Attention will focus on your pretty eyes rather than on your round cheeks. It can't be said often enough: use makeup to emphasize what you *like* about yourself instead of to hide what you don't like.

Still, practice can make for some wonderful and subtle effects with shading and contouring. Especially for the new important evening makeups that we are seeing more and more now, you will probably want to play around with contouring just for the fun of it. The skill you develop may come in handy next time you are having your picture taken or there is a gala holiday party on the calendar.

For contouring on light skin, you can achieve a delicate natural effect by using a deep shade of translucent powder. Contouring dark skin is really a process of highlighting with bright or light colors rather than deepening shadows. Working with cream blush in bright shades is usually more reliable than applying light-colored powder, which can make dark skin look gray.

If your touch is very light, a soft gray-brown eyebrow pencil can be used to contour. You might also practice contouring effects with a foundation. It should be a toned-down, neutralized shade a little darker than your normal foundation, so that it produces the effect of a shadow on the skin, soft and of no particular color.

THESE ARE THE BASIC SHADING CORRECTIONS:

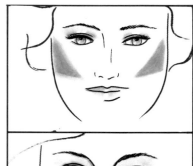

Full cheeks—Draw a triangle with one long side following the lower edge of the cheekbone, a short side near the hairline down to the earlobe and the third side to a point just under the pupil of the eye when you're looking straight ahead.

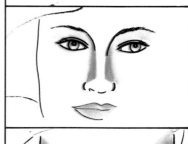

Wide nose—Draw a narrow triangle on the sides of your nose from bridge to nostril. Feather out toward cheeks.

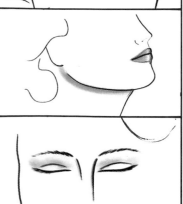

Broad forehead—Shade in a triangle over the brow into the temple.

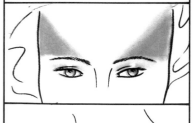

Slack jawline—Lift your head, and shade just under the jawbone.

Long nose—Shade under the tip of the nose.

USING POWDER
LIKE A PROFESSIONAL

When to use it depends on the kinds of products you prefer to use for eye and cheek color. If you like powder blush and eye shadow, then now is the time to complete your makeup base with face powder. If you use creams, liquids and gels for your eyes and cheeks, then face powder comes later as the finishing touch in makeup.

Now or later, be sure to take advantage of powder's benefits. It sets your makeup, helping it look better longer, and does away with shine. Today's powders have nothing to do with the old-fashioned floury ones that were so aging. Powder is nondrying, silky and so microscopically fine it puffs on in an invisible sheen, buffs to a porcelain translucence.

Each model and makeup artist seems to have a favorite trick for working with powder. But in one aspect they all seem to agree: properly applied, a little powder goes a long way. A heavy hand with powder emphasizes lines in the skin.

Getting the most from the least is easy, though, if you use the right tools. Experts choose a soft puff or a fluffy powder brush to apply loose powder. For pressed powder, a clean powder puff or a cotton ball works well.

When you want the most gossamer film of powder: Use loose powder and a powder brush. Dip brush into powder, tap off excess by flicking the brush once against the box. Brush lightly over the entire face, then dust off excess in a downward and outward motion.

When you want a more matte effect and greater absorption: Use loose powder and a puff. Shake out a little powder into the palm of your hand and press the puff into the palm. Pat—don't rub!—powder over your face to press it into the skin. Wait a moment, then lightly buff away the excess.

When using pressed powder: Use the puff in your compact or a fresh cotton ball and dab the cake with it. Shake the puff slightly to remove excess, then gently pat on in the T-zone (the T formed by forehead, nose and chin) and blend downward. The operative word here is "pat," not rub. How often women rub and scrub at their faces with a powder puff! What they're doing is rubbing off all their makeup.

- Deep-toned skins can look gray if powder is too light. Look for translucent powder in deep shades.

- For evening, a very matte finish is a glamorous complement to glittering fashions. Use a pressed powder, patting on gently. Don't rub the puff across your skin.

- Wait awhile before judging the finished effect of powder. For the first half-hour it might look too powdery. Once natural oils of the skin begin to surface, the effect will be more subtle.

- Don't use the same puff to apply both tinted and translucent powders. In fact, using a clean puff each time you apply powder is the ideal way. It's not extravagant if you use cotton balls to apply powder, instead of a puff.

- Use translucent powder to look less tired at the end of a long day. Pat lightly along the outside of your face—across your forehead at the hairline, all along the jawline and chin, and on the tip of your nose. It gives a soft, flattering halo of light.

- For the sheerest translucent glow and to set powder, dampen a cotton pad, squeeze it dry. Then use the damp pad to press lightly all over your face—except your nose, where the matte finish is needed to delay shine.

- Use loose powder to help when you want to blend powder blush. Here's how: Dip a soft powder brush into loose face powder. Blow off the excess; then dip the brush into your powder blush, and brush on with quick strokes. The blush blends into your makeup instantly, with no line of demarcation.

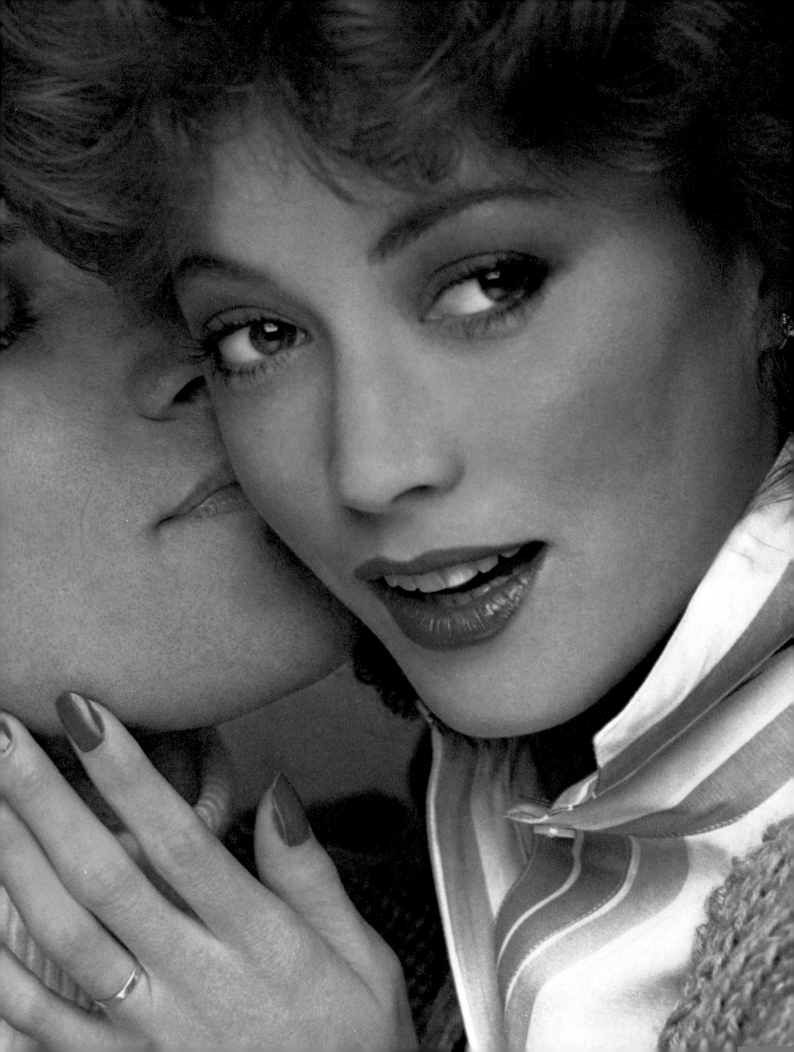

BLUSH

GETTING A GLOW ON

Who can do without blusher? It makes everybody look better: glowing, healthy and alive. Blusher sparks the complexion and makes the eyes look brighter; it's a key to vibrant good looks. Your blusher enhances bone structure as shading and contouring does, yet it's less tricky to work with. Your blusher also unifies and ties together your makeup so that the color on your lips and eyes doesn't have a spotty effect.

TIP—Blush color and lip color should be in the same color family. Therefore you'll need a wardrobe of blush colors to coordinate with your many lipstick shades. It's fun to have a wardrobe of blush colors—tawny ambers, rich winy reds, ripe peaches: a whole range of hues to play with. Experiment with them and you will discover the blush colors that really work for you and make you look as if you were born to wear gray, yellow or any other clothing color you thought you never would look well in.

TIP—Blush that looks too dark in the bottle or compact may be the perfect choice. Try it on, then decide. Blush is concentrated pigment. A color that appears too deep will blend out to a glow on your skin. The real danger is in choosing a too-light shade. Blush color that's too pale just sits there on your skin looking artificial. Dark skins especially need rich, bright blush color. Summer's tanned skin may require a different shade of blush.

PICK THE BLUSH YOU PREFER

■ *Powder blush* produces a soft, matte finish. It's quick and easy to brush on a glow with powder blush, and easy to use when makeup needs touching up during the day. A great choice for normal-to-oily skins. Use it over your foundation and powder. Do use a good, fluffy brush.

■ *Cream blush* (stick or compact) blends to a sheer, natural glow. It glides on over foundation makeup before you powder. Ideal for normal-to-dry skins. For oily skin, there is also oil-free cream blush.

■ *Liquid or gel blush* puts a wash of transparent color over foundation makeup and under face powder.

Frosted blush adds a pearlescent shimmer to your skin. It is available in all forms of blush.
Use it to put glossy color on over your foundation, then blend to a soft luster. Finish with face powder. Great for evening!

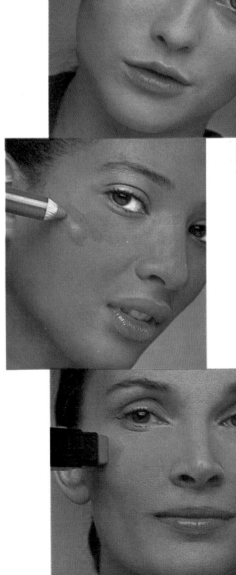

Radiant color! How to glow is up to you. Top, fluff-on powder blush. Center, versatile color pencils. Bottom, handy cream stick blush. All are great for any skin type. Pick what's easiest and most fun to use. Collect blushers in every form and dip into color as the mood strikes.

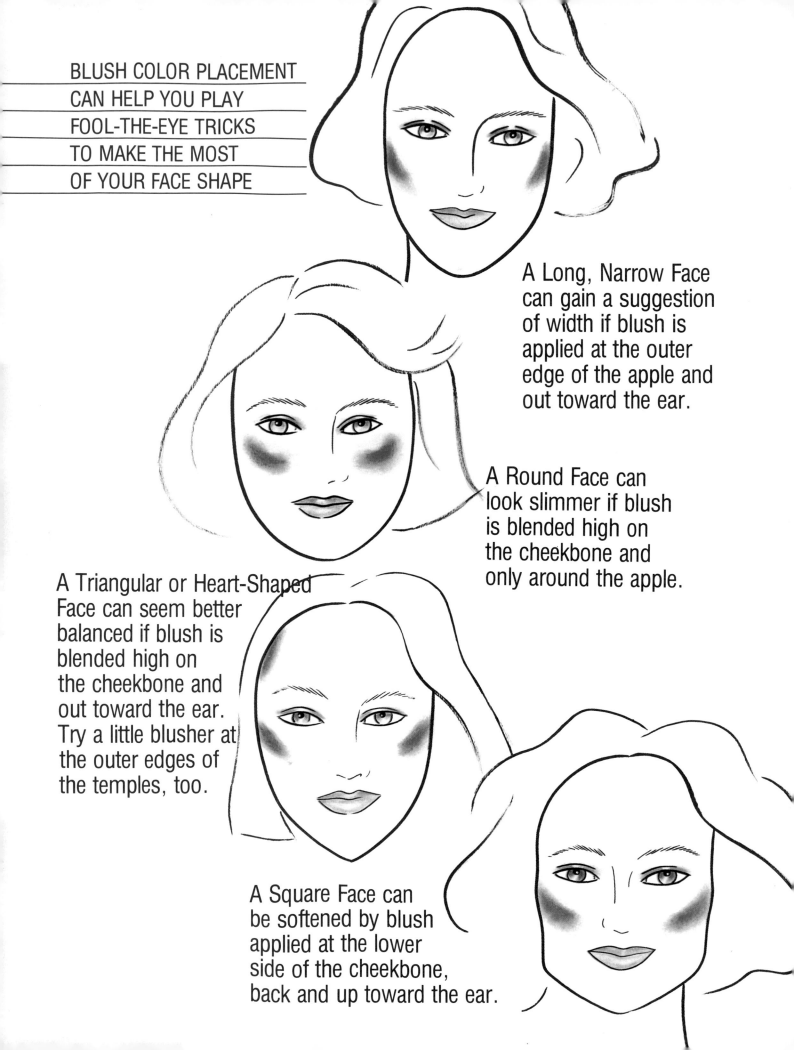

BLUSH COLOR PLACEMENT
CAN HELP YOU PLAY
FOOL-THE-EYE TRICKS
TO MAKE THE MOST
OF YOUR FACE SHAPE

A Long, Narrow Face
can gain a suggestion
of width if blush is
applied at the outer
edge of the apple and
out toward the ear.

A Round Face can
look slimmer if blush
is blended high on
the cheekbone and
only around the apple.

A Triangular or Heart-Shaped
Face can seem better
balanced if blush is
blended high on
the cheekbone and
out toward the ear.
Try a little blusher at
the outer edges of
the temples, too.

A Square Face can
be softened by blush
applied at the lower
side of the cheekbone,
back and up toward the ear.

WHERE DOES BLUSH GO?

That's the most frequently asked question in beauty seminars around the country. The answer is easy: put blush color right where you blush naturally. In case you didn't have a mirror handy last time you flushed with pleasure or shyness, a blush starts right in the middle of your cheekbones, the so-called "apple" of your cheek fills with color, and that's where the blush goes. Of course, you don't have to stop there with blush. A real blush would suffuse with color all the skin that's exposed. You can put a little color wherever the sun would naturally strike your face—across the bridge of your nose, on your temples, at your hairline across your forehead and on the tip of your chin.

VERY IMPORTANT TIPS

- **DON'T** bring color up or in too close to the eyes from below. This makes them look smaller and puffier.
- **DON'T** bring color in too close to the nose. This closes up the face. A good guide is to place your index finger alongside your nose. Bring your cheek color no closer to your nose than the outer edge of your finger.
- **NEVER** bring color down too far on your face. This makes you look drawn. Stop at a point even with the bottom of your nose, or slightly above.

6 POINTERS ON BLUSH

- The deeper your skin tone, the brighter your blush can be.
- Good bones deserve to be accentuated by brighter blush. If your cheekbones are high and chiseled, go bright.
- Party lights, all artificial lights, call for more vibrant blush color. But skip blue reds or purplish tones for evening. Artificial light seems to darken them in an unflattering way.

- To blend cream blush, always tap with fingertips or a damp makeup sponge. Don't rub and tug at your skin.
- For a high-key evening makeup, top off makeup with a quick, light stroke of frosted stick blush just over the tops of your cheekbones for a shimmering accent.
- For a subtle, lasting glow, try layering your blush. First use cream blush; then, after your makeup is finished and you have used powder, apply a little powder blush over your face powder and blend well for a soft, natural color effect.

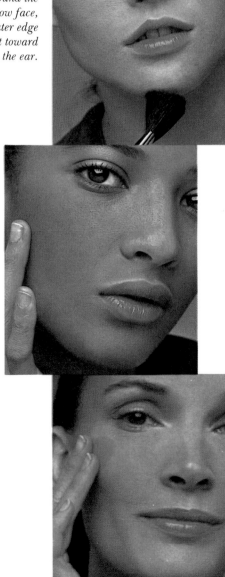

Where to blush? Depends on you—soften angularity, top, with blush high on cheekbone and out toward your ear. Slim a round face, center, blush high on cheekbone and only around the apple. Widen a narrow face, bottom, with blush at outer edge of the apple, blend out toward the ear.

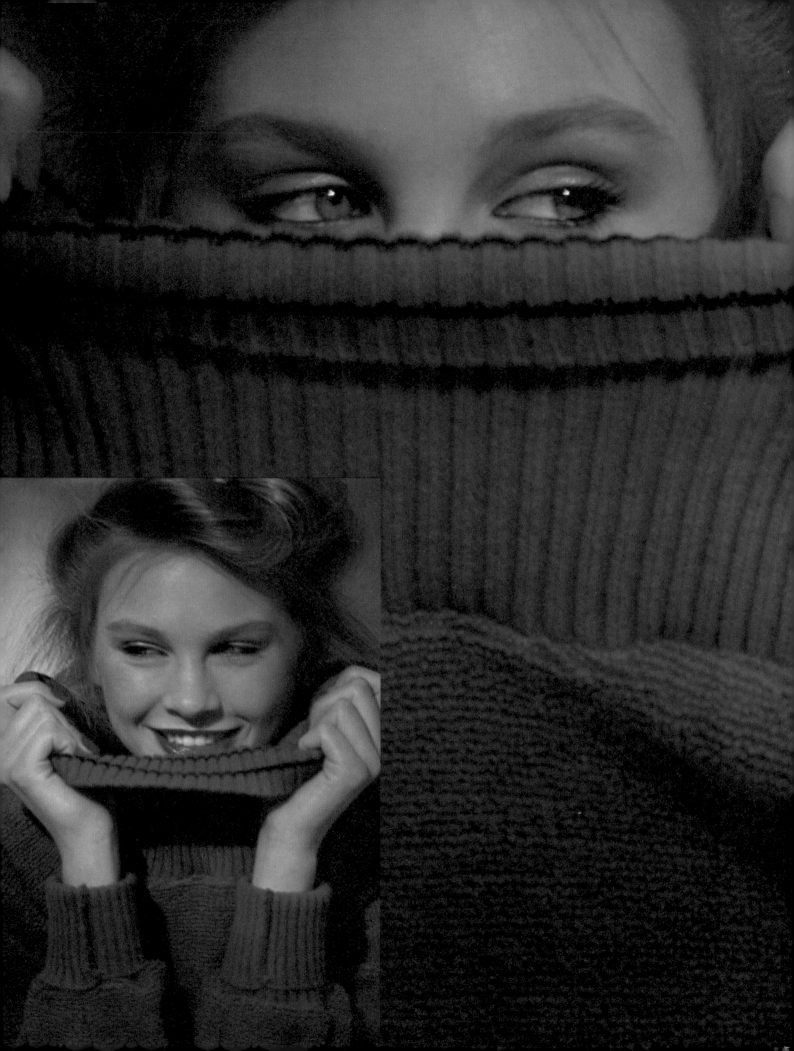

EYES

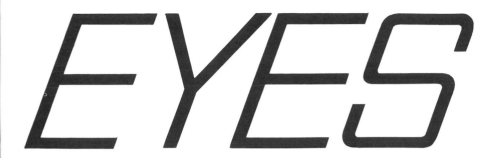

The beautiful first impression you create depends on your beautiful eyes—often the first thing about you others notice. But what they see when looking into your eyes is up to you. With today's makeup and a little practice, you can have eloquent, expressive, memorable eyes.

EYE SHADOW: FOR LIVELY, ELOQUENT EYES

It all starts with eye shadow—shape and color, richness and drama, easy enhancement and fun to play with.

Revel in the fiesta of color for eyes. Use at least two tones—a medium or deep color to shade, a lighter tone to highlight: just one color at a time looks old-fashioned.

Using a blue eye shadow to match blue eyes is another outdated makeup approach. Today we have learned that a complementary color—a reddish brown, for example—will intensify blue eyes by contrast, while a blue shadow will just overpower blue eyes.

Here is a list of just a few of the interesting results you can bring about through using complementary colors for shadows.

EYE SHADOW CHART

Eye Color	Shadow Color	Effect
BLUE	Brown	intensifies blue
	Beige	deepens or brings out gray tones
	Pink	makes blue seem bright, clear
	Plum	deepens, accentuates
GREEN or HAZEL	Charcoal	makes eyes seem greener
	Brown	brings out gold or brown
	Deep blue	makes green clearer
	Pink	brightens the effect of green
BROWN	Blue-gray	all tend to enrich the
	Sage green	depth and warmth
	Plum	of brown eyes
	Lilac	through contrast
BLACK	Plum	all tend to draw attention
	Copper	to the eye and to
	Vivid pink	enliven the eye area
	Deep turquoise	

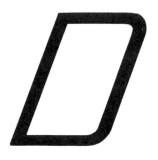**EPENDING ON THE COLORS YOU USE** *to shadow and highlight, and where you place them, you can change the whole dimension of the eye area. Here, in sketches, the game plan. Look it over, then pick the shadow plays that do the most for your eyes*

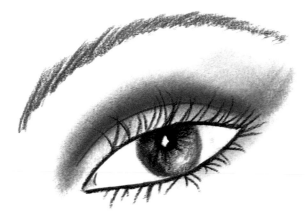

1. To make eyes look LARGER

Sweep color out to the side, along eye bone, under lower lid.

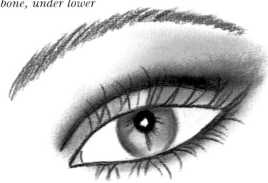

3. To make eyes look DEEPER SET

Put lots of color in the crease. Avoid pale, frosted shades.

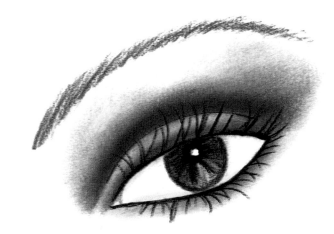

2. To make eyes look FARTHER APART

Sweep color up and out from center to outer corners of lid.

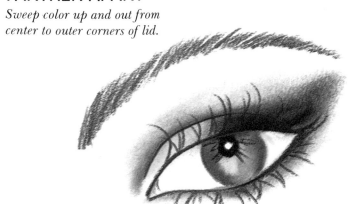

4. To make eyes look MORE OPEN

Shadow all along the lid, lots of color in the crease.

7. To make eyes look LESS DROOPING

Carry color slightly upward at outer corner of the eye. A second shadow color in a lighter, harmonizing shade can be very effective on the eye bone at the outer corners.

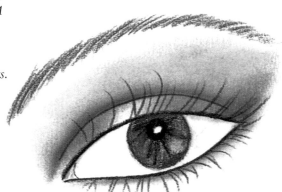

5. To make eyes look MORE PROMINENT

Concentrate color on the eye bone, use a light or frosted shade on the lid.

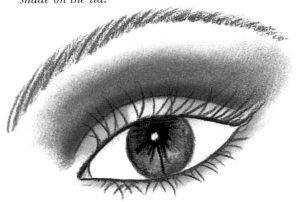

With a little practice you can change the whole look of your eyes. By sweeping the color out to the side along the eye bone (top) you can make your eyes look larger. To make your eyes look more prominent, use more color on the eye bone and put a light or frosted shade on the lid (center) and to make your eyes seem farther apart (bottom) sweep color up and out to the side.

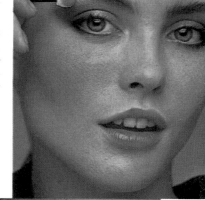

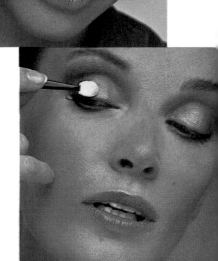

6. To make eyes look LESS ROUND

Shadow the lid only, shading up and out at the outer corner.

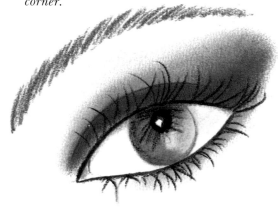

GOOD, CLEAN LINES

Eyeliner is back, and it's nothing like the patent-leather look of the past. You might enjoy experimenting with eyeliner—automatic liquid liner or eye color pencils—during your Beauty Time this week. Although liner is not an absolute basic, many women have discovered it gives their eyes maximum depth and expressiveness and use it for all but the most casual makeup situations. Eyeliner might be just the easy eye brightener you've been looking for.

In liquids and pencils it's possible to draw on the finest, most controlled line if you rest your elbow on a table to steady your hand for maximum balance and control.

Look straight into a mirror with your eyes half closed, lids relaxed. You might want to place the tip of your ring finger at the outer corner of your eye and press gently, slightly toward the temple to hold the eyelid taut.

Draw the thinnest line you can, moving from the center of the lid to the outer corner. Stay as close as possible to the roots of the lashes. Now draw from the inner corner to the center of the upper lid. Lining in two steps this way is easier than drawing one continuous line.

You might enjoy playing with variations on this basic eyelining technique to find the method that's ideal for you.

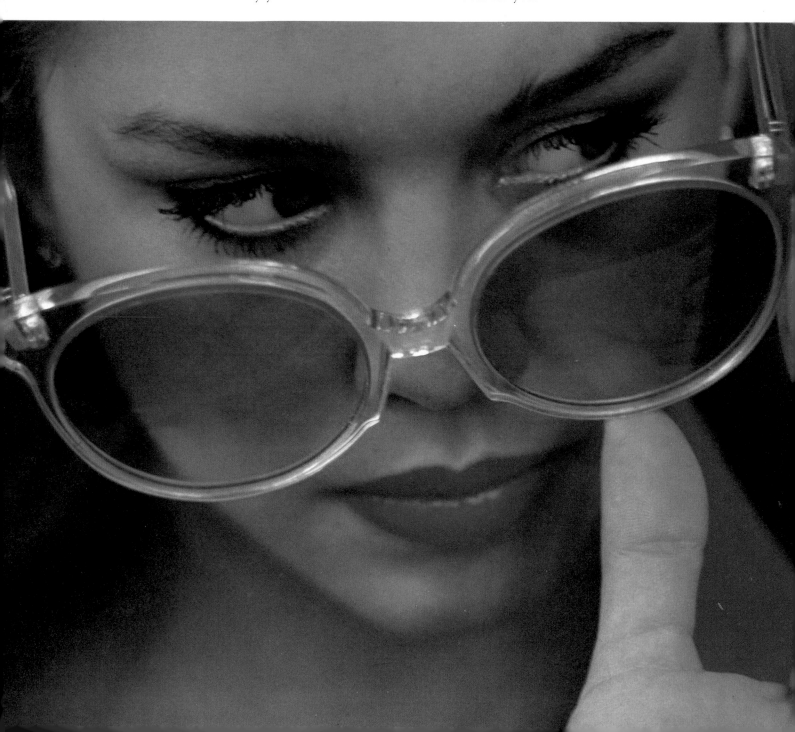

EYELINER VARIATIONS

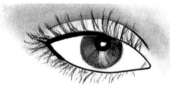

1. *Draw the line just from the center out on the upper lid, and just at the very outer corner of the lower lid, not beyond. Makes eyes look wider than ever.*

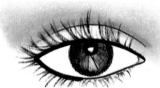

2. *Line the upper lid all the way across. Then line the lower lid from the outer corner to about halfway in. Makes for an extra-intense evening gaze.*

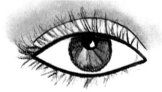

3. *Dot—don't line—just in between lash roots along the upper lid. This takes a little practice, but gives lots of definition and sparkle, without the line.*

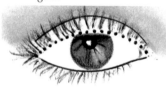

4. *Rim the eye with color by lining the inner lids, top and bottom, with a soft blue or white pencil. Blue all around the inner lids makes the whites of the eyes even whiter; a white line makes eyes look larger; black makes the eyes look very dramatic.*

UPSWEPT LASHES TO OPEN YOUR EYES

Curling lashes before applying mascara opens up the eye. When the white of the eye isn't shadowed by overhanging lashes, it looks clearer, whiter and brighter. A row of upswept lashes helps disguise prominent or puffy eyelids, too. If you wear glasses, curling is a must to keep lashes from sweeping the lenses. Crimp lashes with the eyelash curler, squeezing gently as you slowly count to ten. That's it!

DENSE, DARK LASHES

Now help yourself to wonderful lashes with mascara. Even when you decide to do without any other eye makeup, do curl your lashes and sweep on a little mascara to darken them. Even the prettiest eye looks a little rabbity without mascara, and mascara is the one form of eye makeup that looks good at any age. With just a gleam of eye cream on the lids and lots of lush lashes, your eyes look very young.

Dark brown and black mascara work best on most people.

Automatic mascara, with its bristly little wand brush, or spiral rod, is the easiest to use. Both wands color, separate, even help curl lashes instantly. They are neat, too. If you have a problem applying and get smudges under lower lashes, hold a tissue under them as you apply mascara.

Here's the best way to apply mascara: Do the top side of your upper lashes first. Tilt your head forward, with your eyes half closed. Slowly sweep mascara from base to tips on the top side of the upper lashes. For the underside of your upper lashes, tilt your head back, eyes open wide. To apply mascara to your lower lashes, tilt your head forward and use the tip of the wand.

For extra lushness, let your mascara dry for a minute, then dust a little face powder over your lashes and apply a second coat of mascara. You'll love the extra length and fullness.

TIPS FOR LASHES

- Clumping of lashes comes of rushing mascara application. Go slowly, and separate your lashes with a brush if necessary. Using the tip of the wand eliminates clumping.
- Lashes bleach at the tips in no time when exposed to the sun. Keep them covered with mascara. Try waterproof mascara at the beach. It works!
- Evening makeup trick: after applying one or two coats of black or black/brown mascara, tip your lashes with mascara in a fantasy color—emerald green or sapphire blue.

65

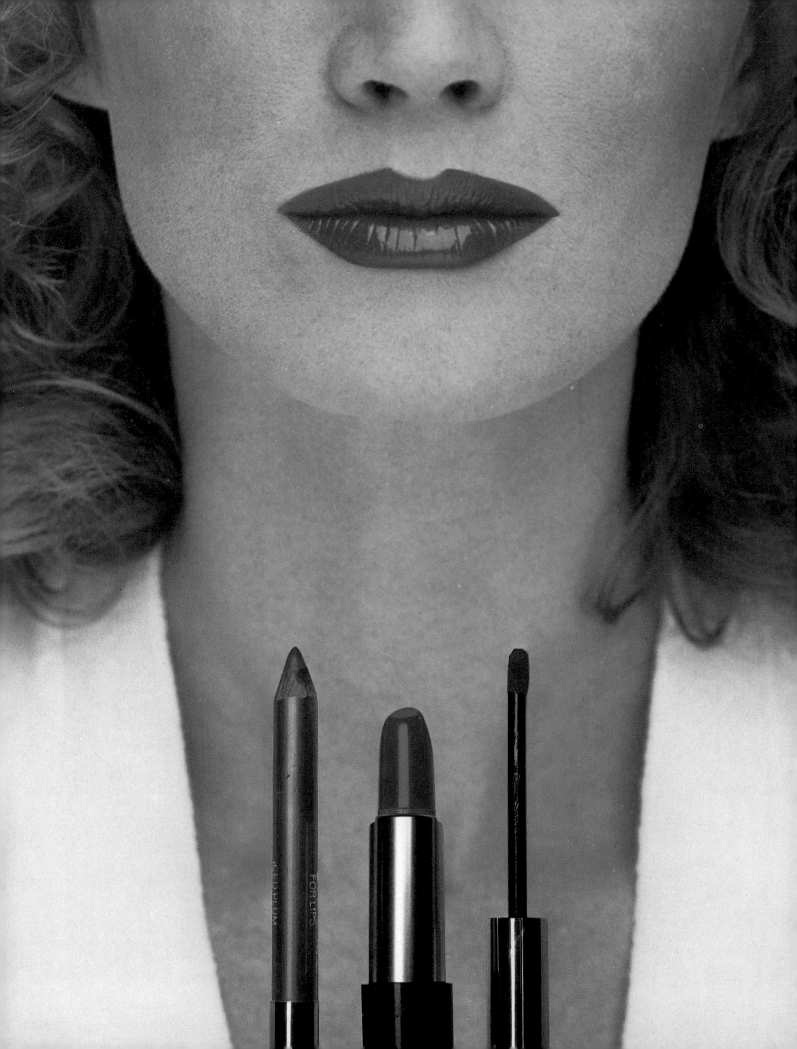

LIPS

Outline the upper lip first, one side at a time. Start in the center of the lip and draw out to the corner in one continuous sweep for the cleanest line. On the lower lip, draw from corner to corner.

2. Color your lips.
Fill in and blend the fill-in color so that it blends invisibly into the outline.

3. Shine your lips
with gloss, clear or tinted, for attention-getting gleam. For a softer glow, omit the finishing gloss. But never blot your lipstick. That not only dulls your lipstick, it robs the lips of color.

To many people, lipstick *is* makeup. Lipstick is the first thing a child grabs when she plays grown-up. In wartime, lipstick has been the one cosmetic governments deemed essential to morale.

No wonder. Lips and eyes are the real focal points of the face; and lips are *the* color accent. Lips communicate, and they do it a lot better with color, shape and shine.

COLOR FOR A BEAUTIFUL MOUTH

To make your lips look moist, sensuous and beautiful:

1. Shape the outline.
You want a clean, smooth edge, not a blurry one. The way to achieve this is by outlining. An outline will also prevent the fill-in lip color you use from "feathering" up into tiny lines along your upper lip. To shape the outline, use a lip brush or freshly sharpened lip-liner pencil. A pencil is more convenient, but it has to be sharp! Keep a little sharpener handy, and use it. If you use a brush, try this balancing act to help steady your hand: keep the pinky resting on the tip of your chin for accuracy and control of the hand.

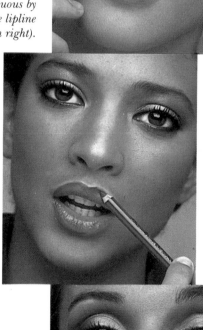

Outline a beautiful mouth. It's step one to sensuous lips. Follow the natural line as closely as possible (top) if lips are shapely. To slim too-generous lips (center) stay just inside the lipline. Make thin lips more voluptuous by coloring just over the lipline (bottom right).

USE COLOR TO CORRECT THE SHAPE OF YOUR LIPS

Perhaps you are less than delighted with a full lower lip or something else about the shape of your mouth. That can be aided by a little color sleight-of-hand. But remember to keep it *slight!*

When you want to redefine lips, bring your foundation over the natural lip line to help conceal it. Then work with your color outline just a hair's breadth over or within the natural lip line. Be very careful to stay just inside or outside the natural line, or the result looks very obviously false.

*for **THIN LIPS**,* draw just over the natural line and fill in with a light or bright color. Finish with gloss.

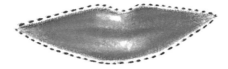

*for **WIDE LIPS**,* stop the outline just short of the natural corners. Fill in the center of the lips with a shade that is slightly darker than the one you use in the corners.

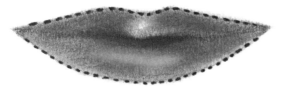

*for **FULL LIPS**,* outline just inside the natural line and stop just shy of the corners. Fill in with a medium or dark color and omit lip gloss.

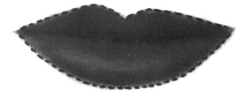

*for **POUTY LIPS**,* use a darker color to fill in the lower lip, a lighter one on the upper lip. Reverse if you want to bring out a timid lower lip. Keep the difference in the shades subtle—just a little lighter and darker—or this trick is too obvious. Omit lip gloss on the lower lip if a pout is the problem, but use gloss if you want to bring out the lower lip.

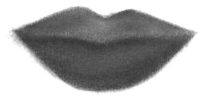

LIP COLOR YOU CAN COUNT ON

For some women, body chemistry can act to alter the effect of a lip color. They find that within a short time, lip color darkens or turns "blue." Many darker-skinned women have· the problem of uneven natural lip color, with the upper lip darker than the lower one.

The answer to these problems is to prepare the lips for color with a foundation, just as you evened out skin tone with foundation. Use your regular foundation, or apply a special lip-toner. Either guarantees lip color that is true and lasting.

15 TIPS FOR LIPS

1. Lip and cheek color need not match, but they should belong to the same color family —warm shades or cool ones together.
2. Make your lips more seductive by blending a tiny dot of clear lip gloss to highlight; place it just at the natural bow of your upper lip.
3. Give the lower lip a pretty suggestion of a pout. Use a dark lip-liner pencil just under and at the center of the lower lip.
4. Always use a brush or lipstick to fill in the color after outlining your lips. When you use your finger to add or blend color, you deprive your lips of all the color and shine that you could have. It all winds up on the finger instead.

lip-lining pencil. Use it just in the curve of the bow on your upper lip, at the center point below your lower lip, and blend it into the gloss.

5. Heavy coats of lip gloss look a little messy. Try a smooth gleam rather than a thick, wet shine.

6. Invent your own color for lips by using a tinted lip gloss over the fill-in lip color you prefer. Play around with various color combinations such as a rich, bright gloss over a soft lip color, or two pales combined, or two brights together.

7. Protect your lips around the clock. Wear lip conditioner to soften and protect lips against dryness and chapping whenever you aren't wearing lipstick. Wearing lip conditioner under lipstick helps keep your lips extra soft and moist.

8. When you want a very delicate, natural look try this: Outline with a very soft, pale shade of lip pencil. Blend well down into the lips using a lipstick brush, but don't add fill-in color. Instead, use a little clear gloss over your lips.

9. Lips need shelter from the sun. Look for a lipstick with a sunscreen. Colorless lip conditioners also come with sunscreens. Be sure to use one.

10. Licking and wetting lips is a bad habit. It robs the lips of color, leads to dryness and chapping.

11. Remove every trace of lipstick color with cleanser at night; then protect your lips with cream or lip conditioner before bed.

12. Unless your teeth are very white and very even, you will find that soft lip colors or rich, muted ones are more flattering than vivid, bright ones. Orangey shades make teeth look yellow.

13. Acidity in food and drink as well as in saliva can produce chemical reactions on your lips that cause the pigment in lip color to alter. Should you find that this occurs with any of your favorite lip colors, use a thin slick of clear lip gloss to protect the true color. And refresh your lip color from time to time with new applications.

14. To make your mouth look very soft and sensual, try using lip gloss just in the center of the mouth on both upper and lower lips.

15. For evening, use a deeper tint of lip gloss to finish your lips. You can also make the shape more seductive by finishing off the usual procedure with another touch of the

Color and shine complete the perfect mouth. You can fill in color after outlining color with a lip pencil, a lipstick (top) or a lip brush (center). Final pretty touch for every pair of lips, the slick of gloss you see going on at bottom right.

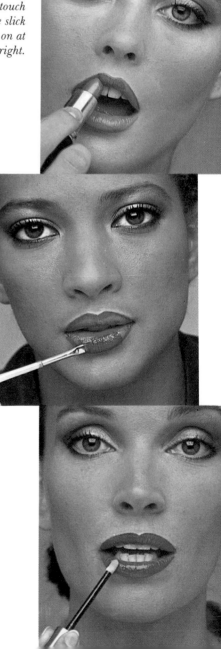

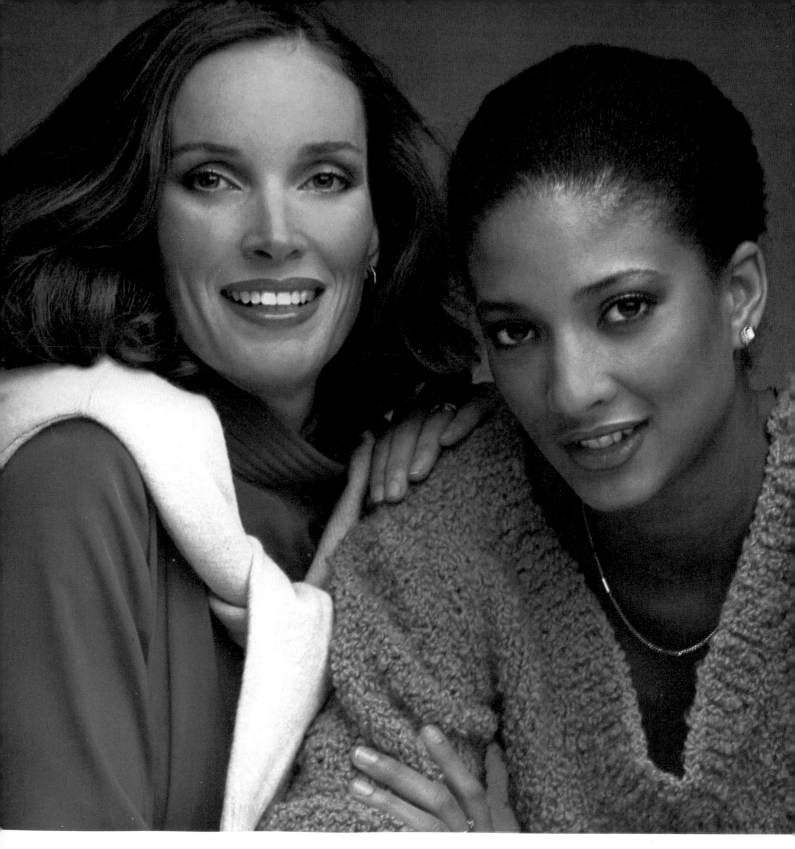

Upbeat good looks, the spark and clean-cut prettiness you see here—that's what it's all about. Making up makes you ready to face the world with all your natural good looks front and center. . . . End results like this are why makeup practice time is well worth spending. These three makeup plans go from naked

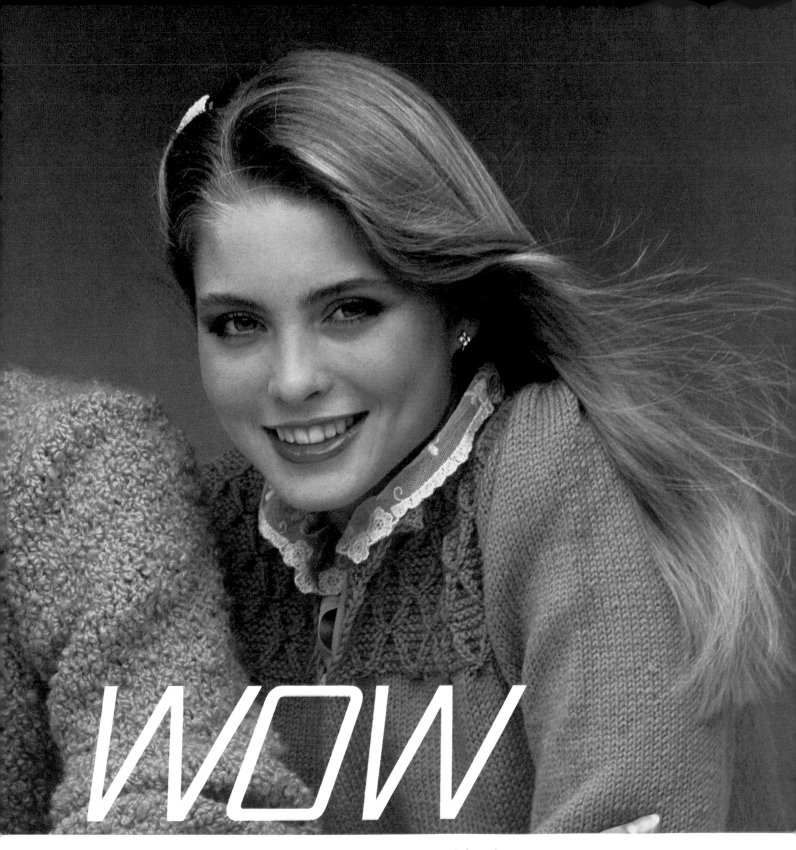

WOW

skin to perfection in well under 15 minutes. Once your own routine is honed and habitual it becomes child's play to do a perfect makeup in minutes, freeing you to get on with your life looking and feeling this assured, this polished, this ready for hours of good times without further thought about good looks.

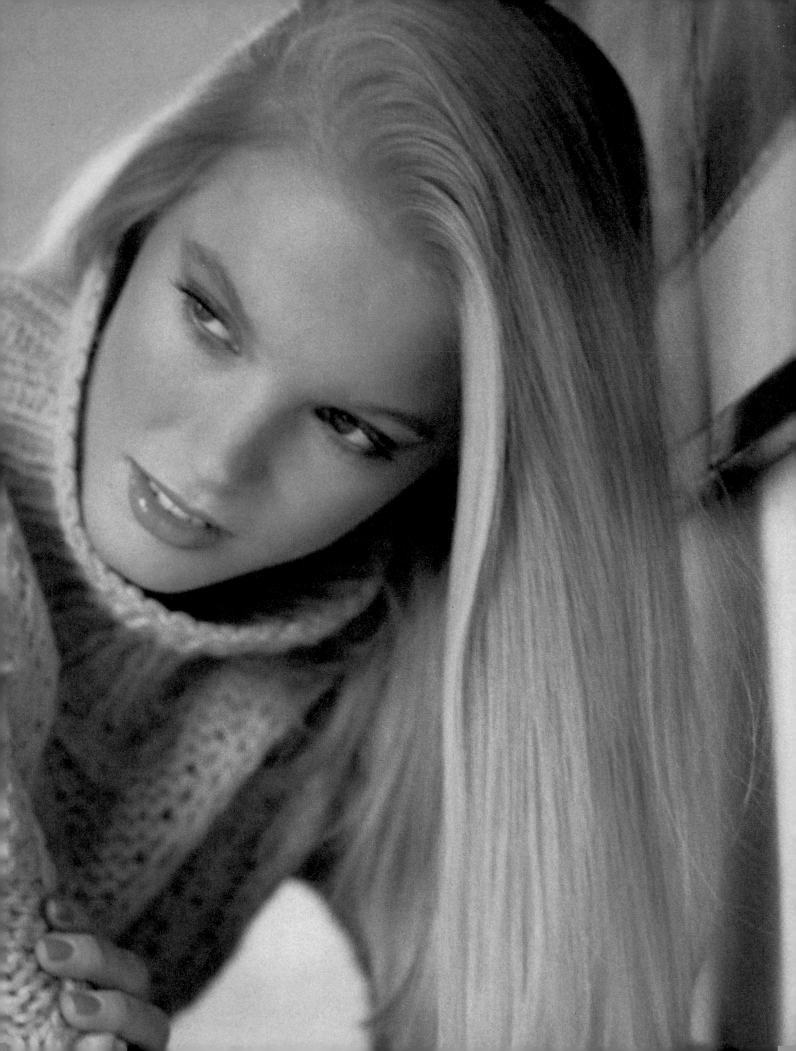

HAIR

Glorious hair

When your hair looks good, you feel happy about yourself, energetic and pretty, even if you're wearing jeans. But when your hair needs a shampoo or a trim, not even the greatest new dress can make you feel attractive. Most women feel that way, but the good thing about hair today is that taking care of it is easier than ever.

Fashion used to demand rigid coifs more suitable to sculpting in stone than to hair, but now we've liberated hair and our thinking about it. Those teased and lacquered bubbles were difficult and time-consuming to maintain if they were to "stay done." But now all of that is in the past, and we recognize that hair looks best when it looks healthy rather than "done." Healthy hair is fat, sleek hair with bounce and shine, hair that looks natural and invites the touch.

On one of the days during your Beauty Checkup, you should give your hair priority: perhaps it will be the beginning of a do-it-yourself makeover, as it is for many women.

After a shower and shampoo, let your hair dry naturally. (Your weekly Beauty Time is the ideal occasion, since you shouldn't be rushed.) While your hair is still damp, use your fingers to comb it back off your face, then let it dry. Once your hair is dry, brush it and then study yourself in the full-length mirror, using a hand mirror to observe all the angles. How does your hair fall naturally? Using your fingers, comb your hair around in different ways. How does it look

swept back or pushed forward into bangs? How do you like your hair up? Maybe you don't have the kind of hair that sweeps around your head like that. If you have very curly hair and have been wearing it long and loose, try pulling it back off your face and get an idea of how you would look in a very short cut, with your hair shorn like a little lamb's fleece. Imagine every possibility.

This kind of playful experimentation is a valuable first step to achieving a trouble-free, super-flattering cut. But of course it is only a preliminary step, a way to liberate your thinking about the style options open to you. The real decision will be arrived at in consultation with your hairdresser, who will give you the invaluable bonus of professional foresight. Only a pro can predict how a cut, a style will work for you.

It often helps, though, if you can *show* the stylist what you have in mind, since most of us are at a loss for words in describing a hairstyle. Before your appointment, go through recent issues of your favorite women's magazines to find a few photos of hairstyles that you like and think will look good on you.

Cut them out, and when you go in to see the stylist for a cut, take them along. Don't be shy about expressing what you want. A good stylist welcomes every clue as to what will make the client look better, because then she will be a better walking ad for the salon. If the pictures you've found are styles that really won't work for your hair, a good stylist will say so. Then the two of you can get down to some creative hair work, coming up with the really unique cut that's designed just for you.

To make it easier, here's what you can do:

■ Select the salon carefully. Look around, and when you see someone with a cut you admire, ask her who cut her hair. If the same stylist is mentioned by several people, go to the salon to have a look at the work done there. No good salon minds a visit from a prospective customer. If you feel timid about just walking in, call first and say you want only to meet the stylist for a consultation. It's often free.

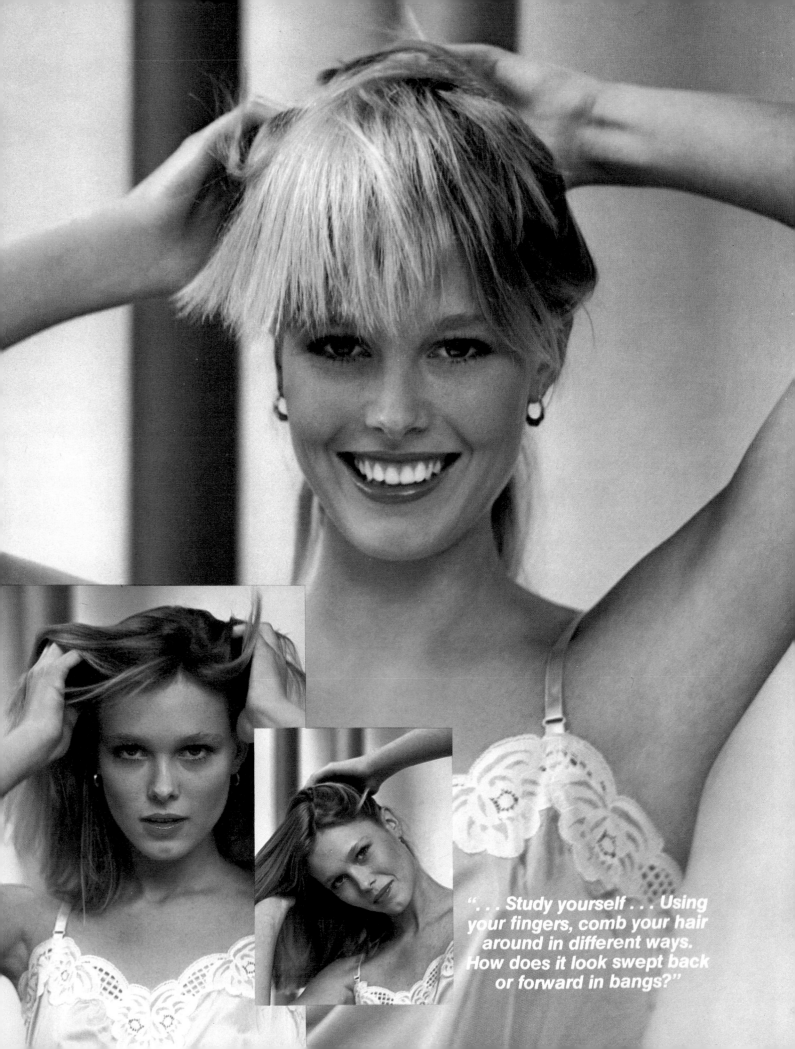

"... Study yourself ... Using your fingers, comb your hair around in different ways. How does it look swept back or forward in bangs?"

- Be honest about what you want from your hair, and how much time you can devote to it. If you are all thumbs at setting, say so. If you want easy, wash-and-wear hair, tell your stylist.
- If the salon seems to give every woman an almost identical cut, the *style du jour,* look further or be prepared to look like a cookie-cutter version of everyone else. But if the work of the salon seems varied and suitable to the women who go there, make an appointment. It could be the start of something beautiful for your hair and your life.
- Ask the stylist to show you several ways to wear your hair with its new cut. Experiment with ribbons, combs; ask him to suggest ways to fix it for very formal occasions, for romantic evenings and for the times when your hair *must* not fall in your face: tennis, jogging, gardening, and the like.

SOME CONSIDERATIONS
ABOUT CUT AND STYLE

- A blunt cut is always healthier for hair, because it leaves only a small area of the ends of the hair exposed. The end of the hair is the most vulnerable to damage, and cutting hair at an angle exposes a long diagonal hair end to moisture loss and damage such as splitting.
- Minimal layering may be necessary to control curly hair.
- Split ends can be eliminated only by cutting them off. If split ends are far advanced, you may need to trim as much as two inches at your next haircut. Once split ends have been eliminated, be very gentle with your hair to discourage splitting.
- A mature face may be flattered by shorter hair, but not by *tight* short hair. Softness around the face is much more becoming to the older woman than severity. Gray or white hair usually looks best if there is a bit of movement or wave away from the face, and looks less good when worn tight against the head.
- A thick neck or a double chin is greatly helped by slightly longer hair curving in just under the jawline.

- Look at all the angles when having your hair cut. Be sure the style looks as good in profile as it does full face, that it's as becoming when you stand as when you sit in the stylist's chair. Stand up; examine the effect in a full-length mirror and with a hand mirror to see the back, the sides and the total effect.

HOW HAIR GROWS

Your scalp is covered with hair follicles—more than a hundred thousand of them—which change protein into hair. You have the greatest number of follicles if you're blond; brunettes have fewer, and redheads the least number of follicles. When you are born, the follicle is tiny and produces a silky, baby hair. But they grow as you do, until along about your twelfth birthday, when they reach maximum size and grow the thick hair of adulthood. Late in life, follicles may shrink in size and produce finer hair, as in childhood. The shape of the follicle determines the look of your hair. Straight hair grows from a follicle that is more or less round in shape. The hair itself is round in cross section. When the follicle curves, the hair is almost kidney-shaped in cross section, and grows out wavy. Curly hair is oval in cross section. It grows from a follicle that is very curved below the scalp and forces the hair into curls.

At the base of each follicle are a tiny muscle, an individual sebaceous gland and a bulb-shaped hair root, nourished by capillaries in the scalp. This root grows at an average rate of one-half inch a month. As it grows, it pushes the shaft of old growth up and out of the way. This dead shaft, pushing up above the scalp, is the hair we see. The living hair is below the skin.

For about a thousand days the single hair keeps growing. Then the follicle rests for about a hundred days. The root stops growing during this rest period, and its attachment to the base of the follicle becomes very loose. Eventually, a new growth period begins and the new hair shaft pushes the old one out of the way (if it hasn't already dropped off) so new growth can take place.

At any given time, about 10 percent of the follicles are resting and the others are in a growing stage. So your scalp is constantly shedding old hair. Up to one hundred hairs a day are shed by a healthy scalp.

SAVE THE ENDANGERED CUTICLE

Just as you have to peel an orange to enjoy the fruit, so some damage to the cuticle—the outer covering of the hair—is inevitable if you are to enjoy your hair. Combing, shampoos, anything that helps hair look clean and neat roughs up the cuticle. Conditioners help solve the problem. They coat the hair shaft to protect the cuticle against weathering and, at the same time, patch up little fractures and peeling cells that are the inevitable by-products of keeping hair in good shape.

KEEP HAIR HAPPY WITH THE BEST CARE

So that hair can thrive, the scalp must be kept in good condition. That means free of dirt, oil and scales of dead cells that would clog the pores and the hair follicles. And the circulation has to be brisk. Follicles depend for nourishment on a rich supply of oxygenated blood coursing through those tiny capillaries. What helps circulation? Yoga headstands and plenty of exercise, of course. But so do lazy, relaxing sessions of scalp massage. This soothes tensions all over, not just in the scalp.

Prop up pillows at your feet, and lie across

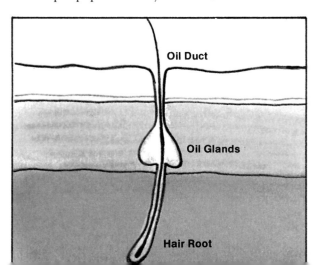

Oil Duct

Oil Glands

Hair Root

the bed on your back, with your head hanging comfortably over the edge of the bed. Using the pads of your fingers, start at the base of your neck and let your fingers crawl up and across your scalp. Use little circular motions. Be firm —you want to really move the scalp around— but be gentle; don't rub or tug at your hair. Massage for as long as you like—say, five minutes—and see how good you and your scalp feel. If your hair is very dry, massage every day if you can. If it's oily, massage before a shampoo. Of course, it's ideal to have someone else massage you. But reciprocate!

BRUSH FOR LUBRICATION

Brushing is relaxing, and doesn't hurt the circulation. But the real purpose of brushing is to lubricate the hair. Brushing distributes natural oils evenly along the hair shaft from root to end, but you must brush slowly from the scalp. Rapid brushing of the ends of the hair only is something you see people doing all the time. It may help to relieve nervous tension, but it doesn't do a thing for hair, except perhaps to hasten split ends.

BRUSH THIS WAY. Bend from your waist and brush your hair forward over your head, from the scalp to the ends. Use long, continuous strokes. Straighten up. Starting with the hair at the nape of your neck, brush your hair down and out. Twist your wrist at the start of each stroke. For more volume, try using two brushes, one in each hand.

That's the way to brush for extra shine. When you're brushing to tidy your hair, you don't have to bend over. But you should still brush from the scalp out to the ends, being careful not to rake the scalp. A good brushing—and a good brush—doesn't scrape scalp or hair.

USE THE RIGHT BRUSH. Your brush should be appropriate to your hair's texture and length. Softer bristles are for fine hair, stronger bristles for coarse, curly hair. Natural bristles are good because they are gentle, and best at polishing hair because they absorb oil and dirt. Synthetic bristles can take tougher treatment, and of course are ideal for use with heat, when blow-drying. Good ones are made so that they're gentle too, with rounder tips that won't harm hair.

Take care of your brushes. Run a wide-toothed comb through brushes to remove hair. Keep brushes scrupulously clean. A dirty brush dirties your hair. To properly wash your brush, fill the basin with warm water and a little shampoo. Dip the brush in and swirl it around to clean it. Don't soak the brush—you loosen bristles—and don't wet the back of a wooden-backed brush. Rinse in lukewarm water. Wipe the handle dry, and let the brush dry, bristles up, on a towel. To speed up the drying, you can set the blow dryer on Cool and play a stream of moving air across the brush. Store a brush bristles up.

You never need count to one hundred strokes when you brush. In the old days before frequent shampoos, women had to brush more to keep their hair clean. Now twenty strokes is more than enough to clean and shine hair, dislodge loose hairs and whisk away surface dirt and hair-spray buildup. If you use hair spray, brush it out every night before bed. Heavy spray makes hair too brittle to sleep on. You should also brush nightly if your hair is dry: brushing helps spread natural oils. Everybody should brush before a shampoo to get oil up and off the scalp for the gentlest and most thorough cleansing. But *never* brush wet hair, or even damp hair. Hair is very elastic when wet, and brushing can pull and stretch it to the breaking point.

Combs are made for maneuvering wet hair. Use a wide-toothed comb to distribute conditioner in wet hair, or to part and section it for setting and drying. A comb with closer-set teeth can be used to comb and groom hair at other times.

The best comb, no matter what it's made of, must be flexible and have blunt, rounded teeth. There should be no sharpness. Test by running your finger along the edges of the teeth. Throw away a comb with broken teeth. Missing teeth on a comb can bite your hair. Keep your combs as clean as your hair, washing them in water and a little shampoo; then rinse well, and dry.

When you comb wet hair, start at the ends of the hair, one small section at a time, to gently untangle—never pull!—and work up to the roots. If your hair, when dry, is excessively windblown, use the same method.

Static electricity sometimes makes combing and brushing difficult. Here's a solution: use a creme rinse or conditioner. It works!

HAIR'S BEAUTY BASIC

Of all the things you can do to make your hair look better, there's one that is basic. Shampoo. Dirty hair is never decorative. Only washing it can uncover the light and shine, the color and swing that are basic to beautiful hair.

How often to wash? As often as you like: at least once a week, or every day if you wish. If you wash every day, use a gentle shampoo. You wash your face every day, and hair goes everywhere the face does, so it gets just as dirty. In fact, it gets even dirtier, because it has more surface and oil to hold on to airborne dirt. It is also more porous, so it traps and holds airborne grease and smells. Some people used to think frequent shampoos wash away hair, but if that were true we could all wash our legs and underarms and forget about shaving. Don't worry about overdrying hair; if you use only the right (small) amount of the correct shampoo and lather only once, your hair will not dry out.

The correct shampoo is something you have to find by shampooing. But there are plenty of clues to help you find the one that's best for you.

Start by narrowing the field to those shampoos which are formulated for the state of your hair. Dry, normal and oily hair all have special formulations. In addition, there are especially gentle shampoos to care for processed or damaged hair.

Consider how frequently you'll use your shampoo. The more often you wash, the less heavy-duty action you need. We all wash our hair more frequently now, and manufacturers take this into account. The newer the shampoo, the less active it's apt to be. A further clue is on the label. If it's gentle or mild enough for a baby, it's right for daily use.

What about pH and acidity? In the face of all the advertising around, this may sound like heresy. But . . . what you should most concern yourself with is a mild shampoo, and even more importantly, with rinsing it all out. Here's why.

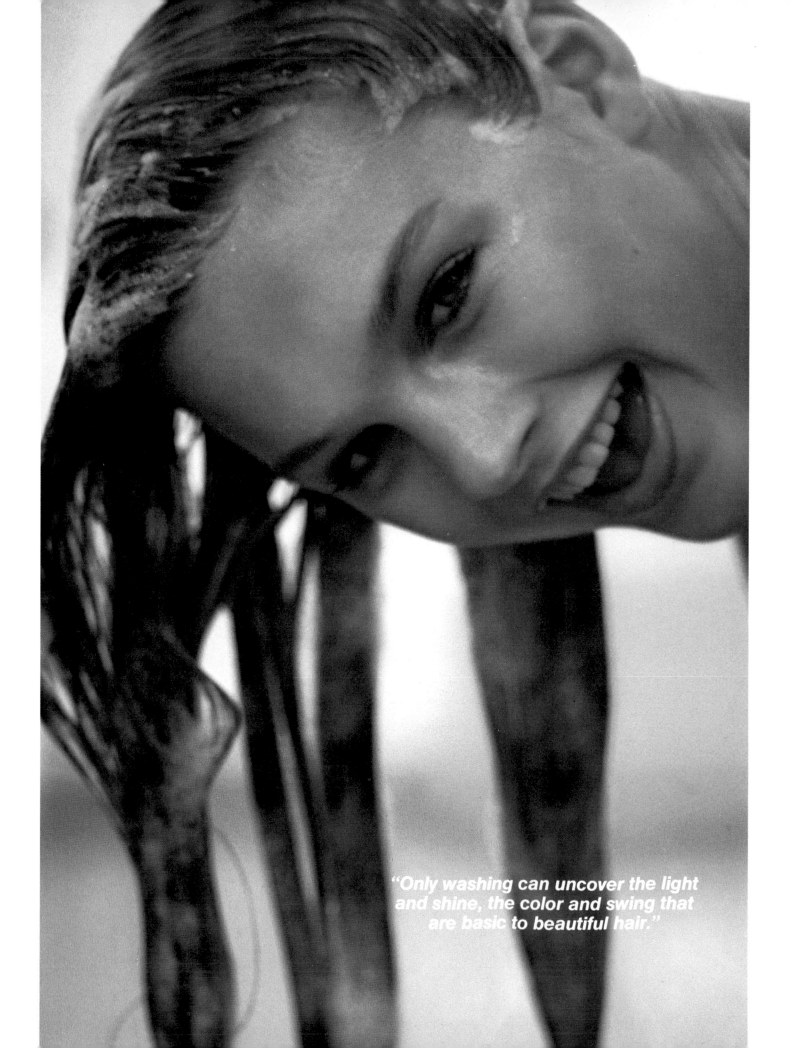

"Only washing can uncover the light and shine, the color and swing that are basic to beautiful hair."

Chemists measure the state of the hair (like the skin) on the pH scale. This scale runs from 0 to 14, with the lowest numbers representing acidity and the highest, alkalinity. A pH of 7 is neutral, neither acid nor alkaline. Healthy hair has a pH reading of 4.0 to 5.0. When hair is immersed in an alkaline solution, it swells and the scales of the cuticle rise.

Soap and water is a highly alkaline solution. If you wash your hair with soap, the hair swells and the cuticle lifts to the utmost. The soap and water washes off the dirt and oils that are on the hair, but it's very hard after washing to remove all the soap. Almost impossible, in fact. So after washing, the hair is coated with a film of soap scum. This alkaline residue keeps the cuticle lifted, even after the hair is dry, so it looks dull and is easily damaged.

So a very acid cleanser would be good for hair, right? Wrong! First of all, the more acidic a cleansing solution is, the less it lathers. In purely scientific terms, it is possible to produce a cleanser for hair that doesn't lather at all. But would you *feel* that your hair was clean? Nobody does. So people just add a little more of the nonlathering cleanser, trying to work up some suds. The result is that they use too much shampoo, rub their hair more than is good for it and still feel that their hair isn't quite clean. An even more crucial drawback is that the super-acid solution will not cause the cuticle to swell enough to allow thorough cleansing of the hair shaft. If the water is hard, and your hair is oily, the picture is even bleaker. Very acid shampoo and very hard water can cause dirt and oil on the hair to solidify through a chemical reaction. They are said to complex. Then a few hours later, body heat melts these dirty solids and they may then coat your hair so that it looks dirty all over again.

What's the solution? A mild, gentle shampoo that is pH-balanced. This is a shampoo with a satisfying lather, a gentle cleansing action, one that's economical to use and easy to rinse off and that leaves your hair in a neutral state. But how do you restore hair to a pH of 4.0 or 5.0? Quickly and easily. With an instant-conditioning rinse to use immediately after shampooing. This conditioning rinse will restore normal pH, and coat the hair shaft to make the hair softer and shinier. A creme rinse may restore normal acidity to the hair, but its real aim is to make hair easier to comb after shampooing and to impart a pleasant fragrance to the hair. If you should happen to run out of creme rinse or instant conditioner, you could restore your hair to natural acidity by using an old-fashioned lemon or vinegar rinse: add a tablespoon of lemon juice or vinegar to a pint of water for the next-to-last rinse. But avoid these homemade rinses if you have had a permanent or your hair has been colored; they can be very drying.

HOW TO SHAMPOO

1. Brush your hair first to distribute oil throughout the hair and to loosen dead cells and falling hairs. Use the shower for easiest, most thorough cleansing. If you have no shower, invest in an inexpensive rubber-hose shower attachment for the bath. It's almost impossible to get hair really clean, thoroughly rinsed in the sink.

2. Use warm water. Wet your hair thoroughly. Throw your head back so that soil rinses out of your hair and runs off behind you, not down your face. This also keeps long hair from tangling.

3. Pour a small amount of shampoo into your wet palm and rub your palms together to work up lather. Pouring shampoo directly onto hair makes even distribution harder. Don't scrub and mush up long hair to work shampoo into it; that tangles hair hopelessly. Comb through your hair with your fingers; then work suds from your scalp to the ends and gently massage your scalp with your fingertips. Massage lather into the scalp and hairline, then work it out to the ends. Be gentle; hair is very elastic when wet and can be damaged by too-vigorous pulling and scrubbing.

4. Rinse thoroughly in plenty of running water. Warm, not hot.

5. Do not relather unless your hair is very dirty or oily. But do rinse again as often as you like. Many hair experts advise that you spend four times as long in rinsing as in washing. Hold your head back while you rinse, especially if your hair is long. As you rinse, gently comb out tangles with your fingers.

6. Hair with rich luster and body, hair that does what you want it to, is the kind of hair that the right conditioner can help you have.

Use an instant conditioner or a creme rinse directly after rinsing out every trace of shampoo. Rinse out thoroughly, as the label directs. *Creme rinses* soften hair that doesn't need more body and may help in setting and styling coarse hair. Some creme rinses are made to be left in the hair to help eliminate tangles, but most are designed to be rinsed out within five minutes.

A conditioning rinse should be poured into the palm, like shampoo, and then applied to the hair. Use on the hair only—don't massage it into your scalp. If the product is to be rinsed out, rinse *thoroughly*.

If you have rinsed your hair thoroughly, it should look very shiny after conditioning, even while it is still wet. If your hair looks dull, there's too much conditioner still on the hair, so rinse again.

PUT HAIR IN PEAK CONDITION

There are also conditioners designed for helping repair hair that's been damaged by the weather or by chemical processes. These intensive conditioning treatments are sometimes accompanied by the use of heat to obtain really penetrating results within a ten- to thirty-minute period. If your hair isn't all you'd wish in the way of suppleness and luster, investigate intensive conditioning-treatment products.

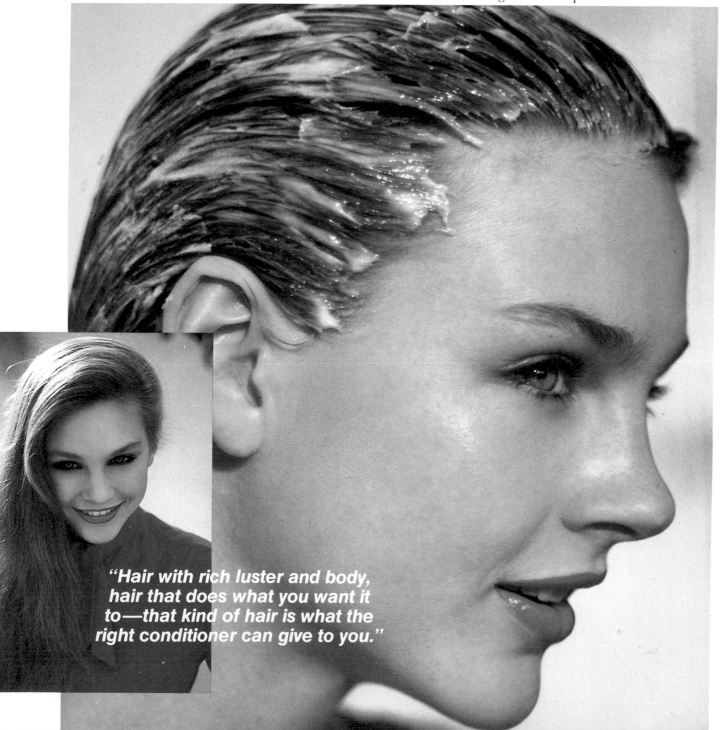

"Hair with rich luster and body, hair that does what you want it to—that kind of hair is what the right conditioner can give to you."

EASY DOES IT WITH DRYING

Here's the gentlest plan to dry your hair after rinsing. Untangle by using your fingers to separate. Start at the ends. (This should be easier if you rinse with head back.) Press palms flat against the head and the hair to gently squeeze out excess water.

Wrap a dry towel over the hair. Let the towel blot hair dry. Don't rub. When moisture has been absorbed, uncover your hair.

Shape and separate hair with a wide-tooth comb. Allow hair to air-dry for as long as is convenient before styling and blow-drying.

HEAT AND HAIR

The plain and simple truth is, heat is not good for hair. But so many of the tools and techniques we use to make our hair look good depend on heat. You can use heat and still protect the health of your hair if you condition regularly and don't overdo the hot stuff.

At very high temperatures, the hair can be damaged. In blasting heat, hair can lose elasticity and strength, along with sheen. Conditioners, which usually contain fats and oils, can melt down and lose sparkle if the heat is too intense for too long.

Keep your blow dryer on the Cool or Low setting as much as possible, and keep it moving around as you dry your hair so that you don't overheat. Hold it away from the hair, too. Air currents are strong, and even twelve inches from your head is not too far for efficiency. It's also better for your hair.

Many hairdressers now agree that you shouldn't blow-dry every day if you can help it. Check with your stylist about a cut that will spring into shape with air drying. Many of the short styles today don't really need hot curlers or blow dryers to look good. Of course, that doesn't mean that you shouldn't blow-dry. Just don't overdo it.

A LIST OF TIPS: Getting
Professional Results
with the Blow Dryer

■ Your hair should be damp-dry before you begin. Towel-dry it first; separate it with your fingers; then use a wide-toothed comb to remove tangles and to make drying quicker and easier.

■ Begin drying at a higher setting, then switch to a lower one when the hair is still somewhat

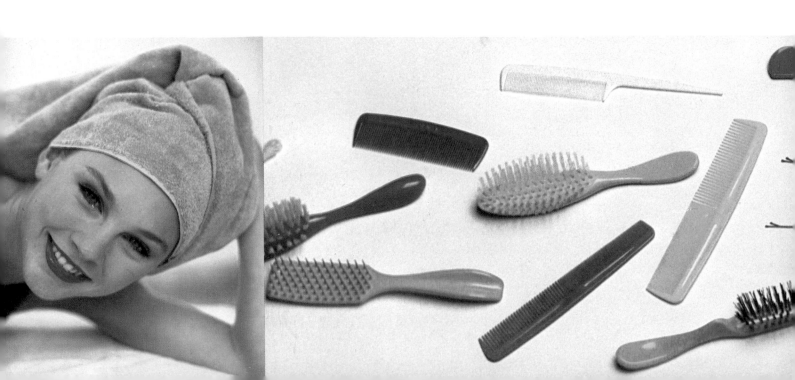

damp. If your dryer has only one temperature setting, or one speed, hold it slightly closer to your hair—about six inches—when you begin to dry, and slightly farther away —eight or nine inches—as the hair dries.

■ Always hold the dryer at least six inches away from the hair, and keep the dryer in motion so that hot air isn't directed at just one spot. Concentrated heat in just one spot can damage hair.

■ Styling as you dry is possible with a round (bottle) brush with heat-resistant nylon bristles. You need a larger brush if your hair is long or thick, a smaller one for short hair. Be sure your hair is almost dry before you start using the brush. Styling with the brush gives hair a much softer and more natural look than it could have if you had put it in rollers and then dried it.

■ Section your hair before you begin to dry it. Use a wide-toothed comb and part the hair into the following sections: sides, sides front, sides back, back, and top front. Dry one section at a time—sides first and top front last.

■ For more volume, part the hair into small sections and use the dryer and styling brush against the natural growth pattern.

■ For fullness, hang your head forward, so that your hair hangs upside down while you use the blow dryer. When you flip your head back, your hair is full and neither flat at the scalp nor poking up in the artificial way that rollers produce.

■ For smooth hair, direct the air current from the dryer down from above and brush the hair downward with long, smooth strokes.

■ For straighter hair, use the brush to grab the ends of your hair; then twist the brush downward so the hair is held taut. Direct air across the top of the hair. Work slowly all around the head to gently stretch each section of hair.

■ To turn your hair under, use the brush to twirl the hair from underneath. Roll the brush down and under. Aim the dryer under the brush.

■ For a flip-up, twirl the hair around the brush from above, sliding the brush down through the hair and rolling it upward at the ends. Aim the air flow up from under, and over the hair on the brush.

A NOTE ON HEAT LAMPS
AND ELECTRIC HOT COMBS

Many of today's shorter styles look best when you use a dryer that does not blow the hair. A heat lamp might be ideal for your look, particularly if you wear your naturally curly hair in a short curly style. An electric hot comb might be the ideal drying tool if you have a short style and straight or wavy hair.

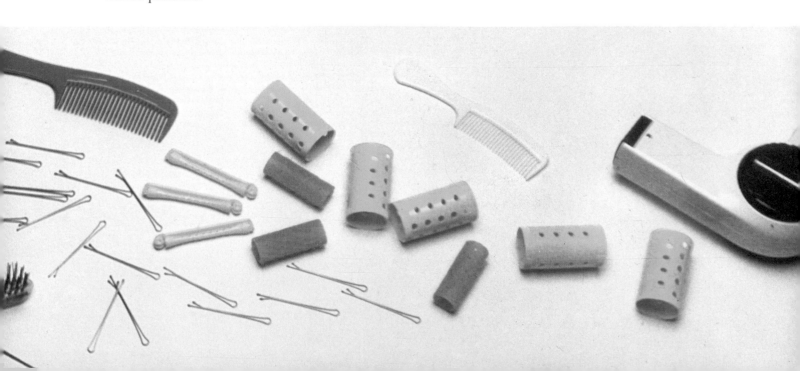

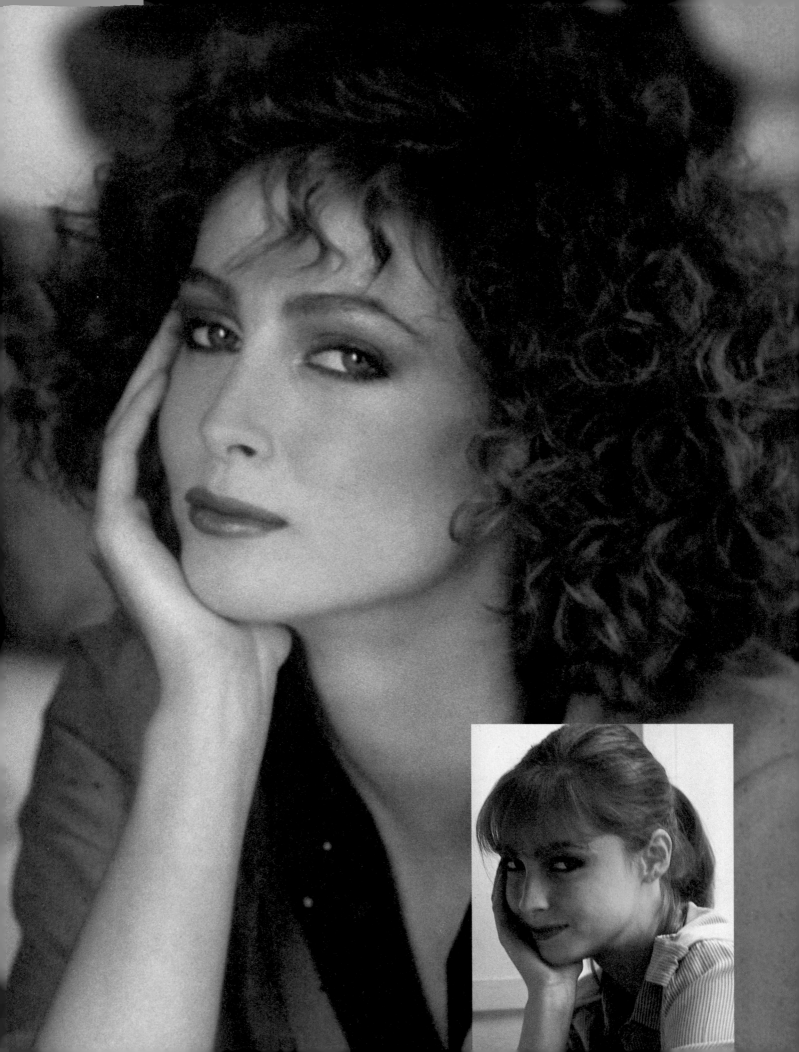

Hair changeovers

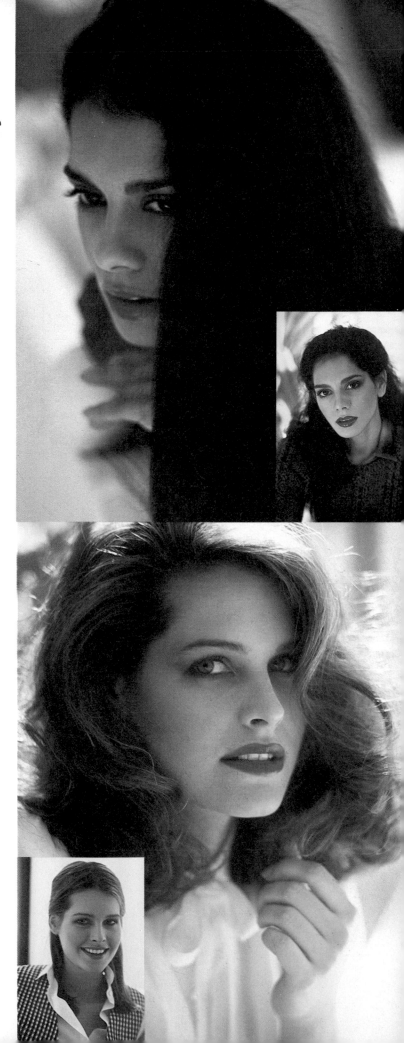

TO STRAIGHTEN HAIR, WAVE IT OR CURL IT

A Permanent can curl hair into ringlets, or merely add waves and fullness. It works by changing the shape of the hair into an S shape that's tight for curls, loose for waves. Hair is wound around perm rods (small rods for tight curls, big ones for waves) and a lotion is applied which releases chemical bonds that hold the hair in its natural shape. It is left on the hair for an exact period of time. Follow the package directions carefully. Then a neutralizing solution is applied to the hair to lock the new shape into the hair. This solution is then washed out, and the permanent is complete.

Your hair should be in good condition before a permanent. You might need one or two conditioning treatments beforehand. After the permanent, wait at least three full weeks before coloring your hair. Always use shampoos and conditioners made for dry or processed hair after having a permanent.

Straightening is a process similar to a permanent. A cream or lotion to break down and soften the hair shaft is applied, then rinsed out, and a neutralizer fixes the straightened shape.

Before straightening, and after, plenty of deep-conditioning is advisable. Straightened hair should be treated very gently.

Don't attempt to combine straightening with hair coloring. It can be disastrous. One model, who both streaked and straightened her hair, got up one morning and found that all her streaks had stayed in bed. The straightened, streaked hair had fallen out and was lying all over her pillow!

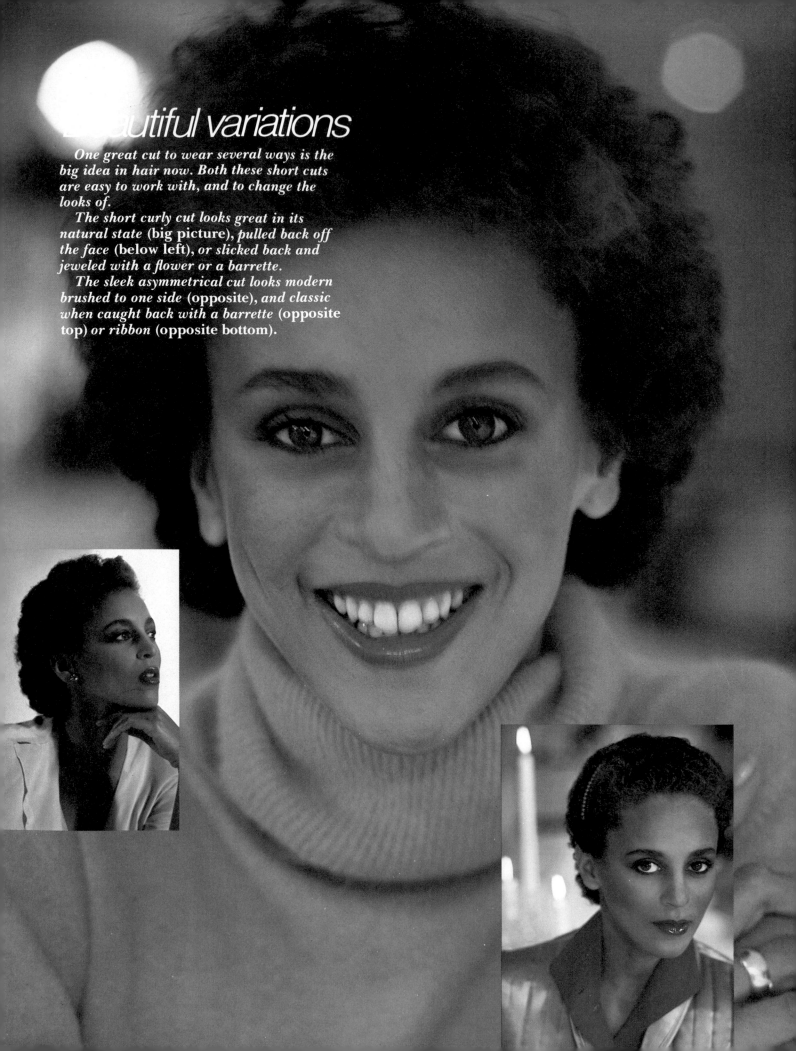

Beautiful variations

One great cut to wear several ways is the big idea in hair now. Both these short cuts are easy to work with, and to change the looks of.

The short curly cut looks great in its natural state (big picture), *pulled back off the face* (below left), *or slicked back and jeweled with a flower or a barrette.*

The sleek asymmetrical cut looks modern *brushed to one side* (opposite), *and classic when caught back with a barrette* (opposite top) *or ribbon* (opposite bottom).

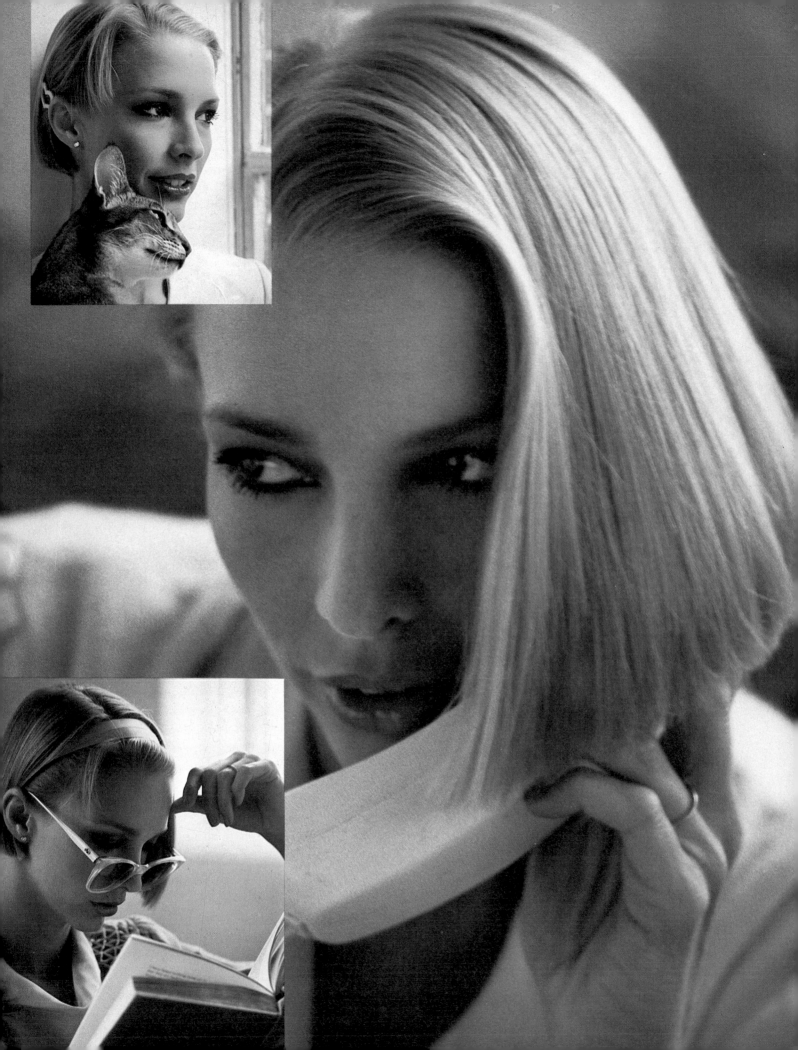

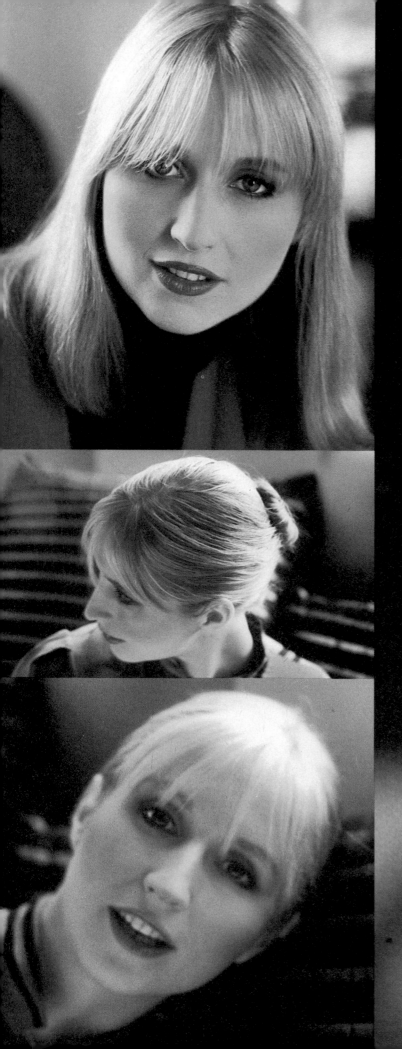

Beautiful variations

Long hair invites playing with—it can be worn up, down, any way you choose. Even with versatile long hair, though, a great cut (to shape, to snip off dead-looking ends) and good care and conditioning make hair easier to work with and prettier.

Left, ways with long hair and bangs: long and gleaming, or pulled up into a neat, sleek twist.

Opposite, from classic modern beauty to romantic traditional beauty with just a few minutes, a few hairpins—that's the allure, part of the lasting appeal of long, long hair.

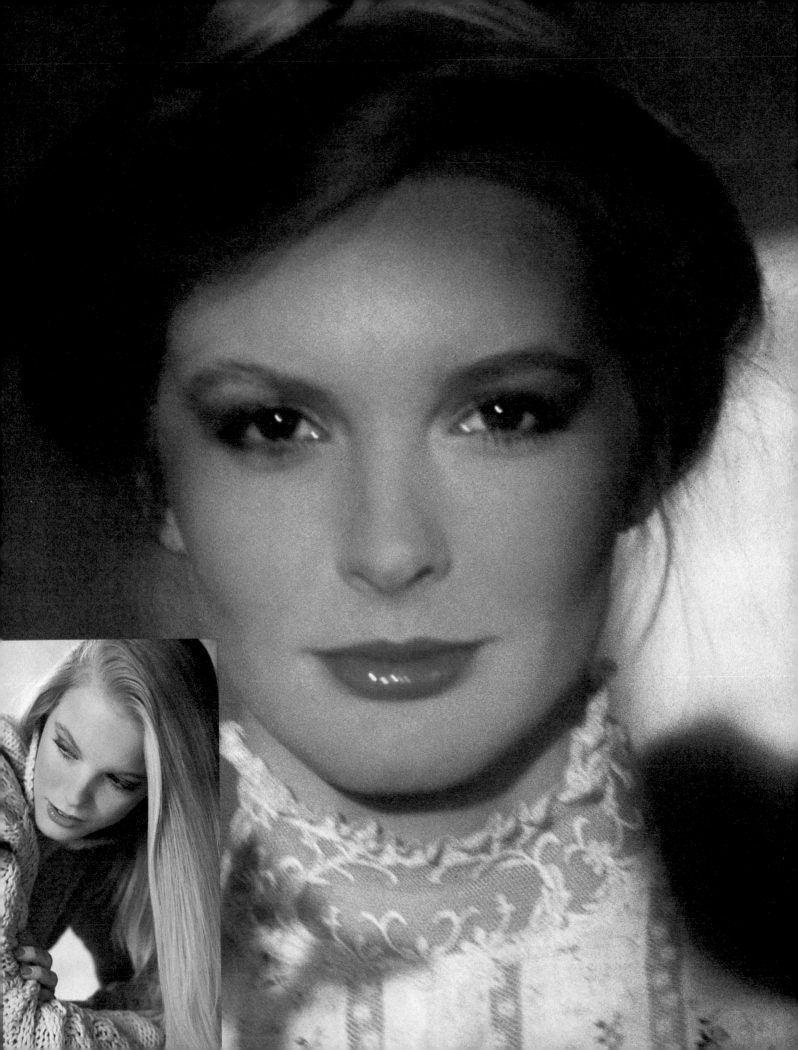

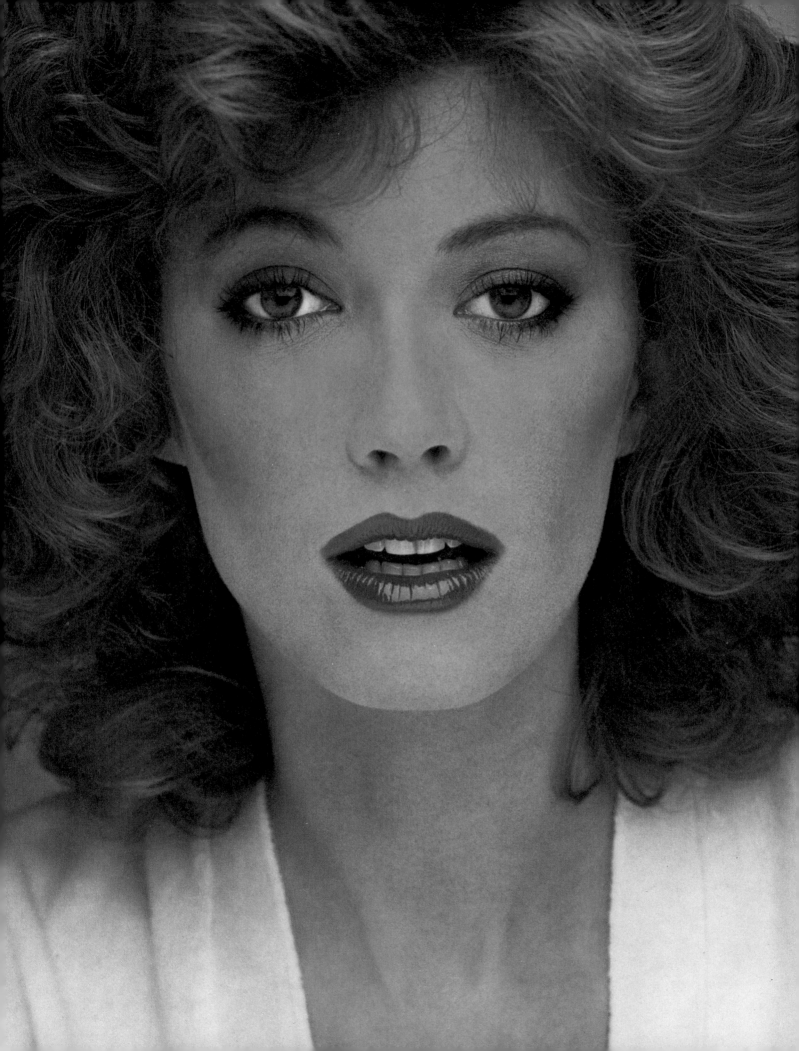

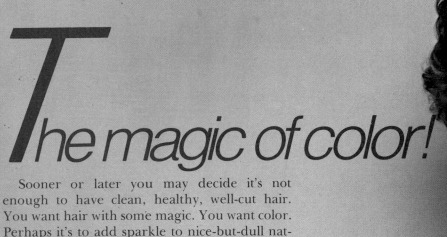

The magic of color!

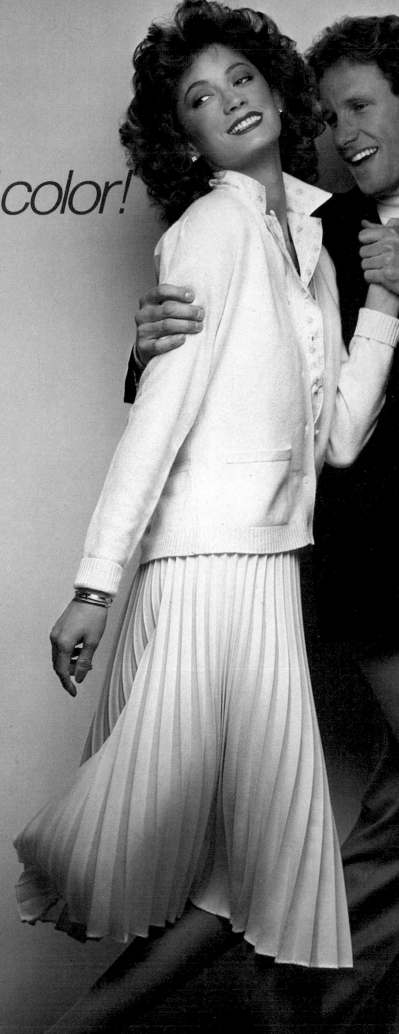

Sooner or later you may decide it's not enough to have clean, healthy, well-cut hair. You want hair with some magic. You want color. Perhaps it's to add sparkle to nice-but-dull natural color; perhaps it's to enhance or cover gray. Well, it's getting prettier all the time. Easier, too. Now even do-it-yourself hair coloring can be safe and subtle.

Subtle is a big word in hair color. Many women shied away because they didn't want a dramatic color change that would force them to become slaves of the touch-up. Hair coloring doesn't have to be like that anymore. That old drastic-change business was harsh and unflattering. The most flattering new color is one no more than one or two shades away from your own natural hair color. This slight, subtle shift of color emphasis can be enough to give you a vibrant new image, but because there is so little contrast with natural color, new growth is very unobtrusive. If you're a week, or even a month, late for a touch-up, it's okay.

Top professional colorists use colors, plural —not just a single color for a head of hair. Hair that's all one color is unnatural and looks it. A blond child's hair may look like a pale-yellow cap, but if you study it up close you can see individual strands that range from palest platinum blond through honey blond to soft ashy brown. Together, they blend into a shimmering overall blond. Good hair colorists today aim for that same lively come-and-go of color in their work.

Another tactic of the professional colorists is to color hair selectively. Rather than changing the color of hair all over the head, the colorist might work with only a few strands here and there to frame the face unobtrusively with brighter hair, as if the sun had struck it. Color is used in streaks, tipped in, painted on just here and there, and swept through the hair. This kind of come-and-go color lets you pick shades that, because of your skin tone, would be unsuitable or unflattering for overall color. As highlights and lowlights, though, they recast the color direction of your hair in a becoming new way. The initial cost of a good professional high-lighting job is usually higher than for an all-one-color treatment. But because you don't require as frequent return visits for touch-ups (usually only two or three a year), it's cheaper in the long run.

Coloring can even help hair's condition. Every color product now has built-in conditioners that may make hair look shinier, feel thicker and be more manageable. Permanent coloring products give hair more body. They open the cuticle so that color can penetrate and swell the cortex. Other chemicals then lock the color into the cortex and reseal the cuticle. The swelling of color gives body to fine hair and can also make a coarse hair shaft sleeker for greater manageability.

COLOR: THE PROCESSES

They range from temporary rinses, which coat the hair with a hint of color that washes away with the next shampoo, all the way to permanent color that's locked in to last. All are available for home use. Color is a powerful tool, however, and the more color you want, the more care you should take. Seriously consider having professional treatment for any permanent color change. The results can outweigh the cost. Only a pro is skilled (and objective) enough to give you all the benefits of color with guaranteed results.

ADD TEMPORARY COLOR

with rinses that coat the surface of the hair shaft with color. These usually contain conditioners, and perhaps a setting lotion. Rinses do not affect the structure of the hair shaft, and are washed away with the next shampoo. Because temporary rinses contain no peroxide, they will not remove color or lighten hair. The color effect is slight, especially on darker hair, but rinses can deepen and enrich color, add glints and highlights. They don't cover gray, but by adding a little color to gray hair can help tone it in.

ADD SEMIPERMANENT COLOR

with no-mix color lotions that slightly penetrate the surface of the hair shaft to add color. Conditioners are built in to add sheen and body as well as color. No peroxide or lighteners are involved, so these products will not remove color or lighten. They will make a more dramatic color change than temporary rinses, will deepen and enrich color and will cover gray. They need no immediate retouching, but the color does wash away after three or four shampoos.

CHANGE COLOR WITH SINGLE-PROCESS PERMANENT COLOR

with shampoo-in or cream-formula permanent color. These penetrate the hair shaft and change its structure with agents (usually 20-volume hydrogen peroxide) that remove the hair's natural color and make it more porous, thus bulkier. These permanent hair colorings then penetrate the hair shaft and deposit a new color. They do lighten hair and do cover gray. The color change is moderate, but permanent. You can cover gray, or you can change your hair to a color that is several shades lighter. In this process, color is shampooed into the hair, or applied with a swab or brush. Just before application the color, an oxidation dye, is mixed with the developer, or bleach (usually peroxide). The color develops when it oxidizes on your hair. And the color lasts until it grows out. This is called single-process coloring because only one step, or process, is involved.

CHANGE COLOR WITH DOUBLE-PROCESS PERMANENT COLOR

with pre-lightening done in one stage and followed by coloring, or toning, to the desired shade. Complete changes of hair color, from dark brunette to pale blond, for example, are possible only with double-process coloring. But the trickiness of the timing and other factors involved make it a job for professionals *only*. Remember too, frequent and regular touch-ups are a must when natural color has been dramatically changed.

THE BLACK WOMAN AND HAIR COLORING

A Black woman's hair can be pure jet black, but it rarely is. Black hair comes in a wonderful wide range of tones from tawny to ebony. Most often, though, it's a very dark, almost-black brown. If you choose to deepen the color to black for drama, or to play up the brown or reddish highlights that may be there, or even if you choose to lighten your hair just a little for a softer effect, that's fine. But be very careful. Black hair is much more absorbent, more porous than Caucasian or Oriental hair, so coloring products are much more difficult to control when used on Black hair. If you are considering any semipermanent or permanent color, it's best to see a professional.

TIPS ON HAIR COLOR

When choosing a color, remember—

■ Pigment in hair and skin are closely related, and both skin and hair become less vivid in coloring as we age. That's why it's a mistake to try to duplicate the color your hair was at sixteen when you begin to color it twenty years later. Brunettes, especially, will find a somewhat lighter shade more flattering. Blondes will probably find a less-bright shade is more becoming.

■ Medium contrasts between skin and hair are always more natural to the eye than high contrasts. If the contrast is too dramatic, the result is ridiculous—for example, the fair-skinned blonde who dyes her hair jet black, or the dark-skinned woman who lightens her hair to silvery blond.

■ Redheads and dark brunettes should be wary of going blond. Be aware of the touch-ups that will be needed very frequently. For best results, stay with a lighter shade of your natural color, and add blond highlights.

■ Streaking, frosting, highlighting and tipping all involve minimal maintenance, usually a touch-up from two to four times a year.

■ Hair color charts usually show a shade as it appears on white hair. Allow for the difference your own color will make when considering how the shade would look on your hair.

■ Wigs can be helpful in judging the effect of a new hair color. Try on wigs in various shades of a color before you decide on coloring your hair.

If you decide to color your hair at home—

■ Test before you color. A patch test, twenty-four hours before coloring, is a must. A small amount of the product is dabbed directly on the skin, in the bend of the elbow or other inconspicuous spot. Next day, check for any sign of skin irritation, and if there is none, proceed to color. A strand test should be used to show beforehand how the color will look. Snip off a bit of your hair, select a strand from underneath, and color it with the product.

■ Pick a time for color when you are rested and relaxed, unlikely to be interrupted. Read the directions over several times and follow them to the letter. Don't watch TV or talk on the telephone during the coloring process. Have a clock handy, or a kitchen timer. Precise timing is important in working with chemicals.

■ Allow at least three weeks between coloring and any other chemical processing of hair, such as a permanent or straightening.

AFTER COLOR—

■ Let a day or two pass before you pass judgment on the color. Natural oils need time to come up in the hair again after coloring, and they make a difference in the effect.

■ Treat hair gently after coloring. Use shampoos and conditioners for processed hair. Avoid using too much heat. Use mist curlers rather than dry heat. Stay out of the sun as much as possible, and wear a cap, scarf or straw hat on the beach. Wear a swim cap in the pool. Rinse your hair with clear water after swimming or sports, and shampoo and condition it when you get home.

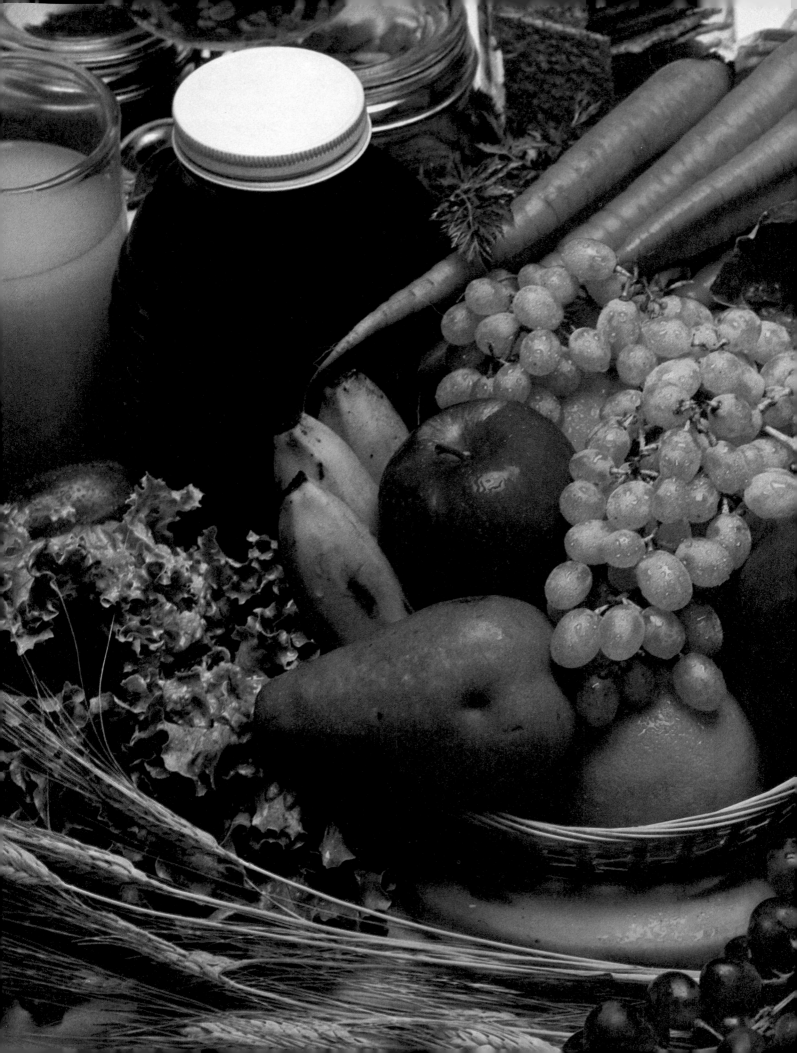

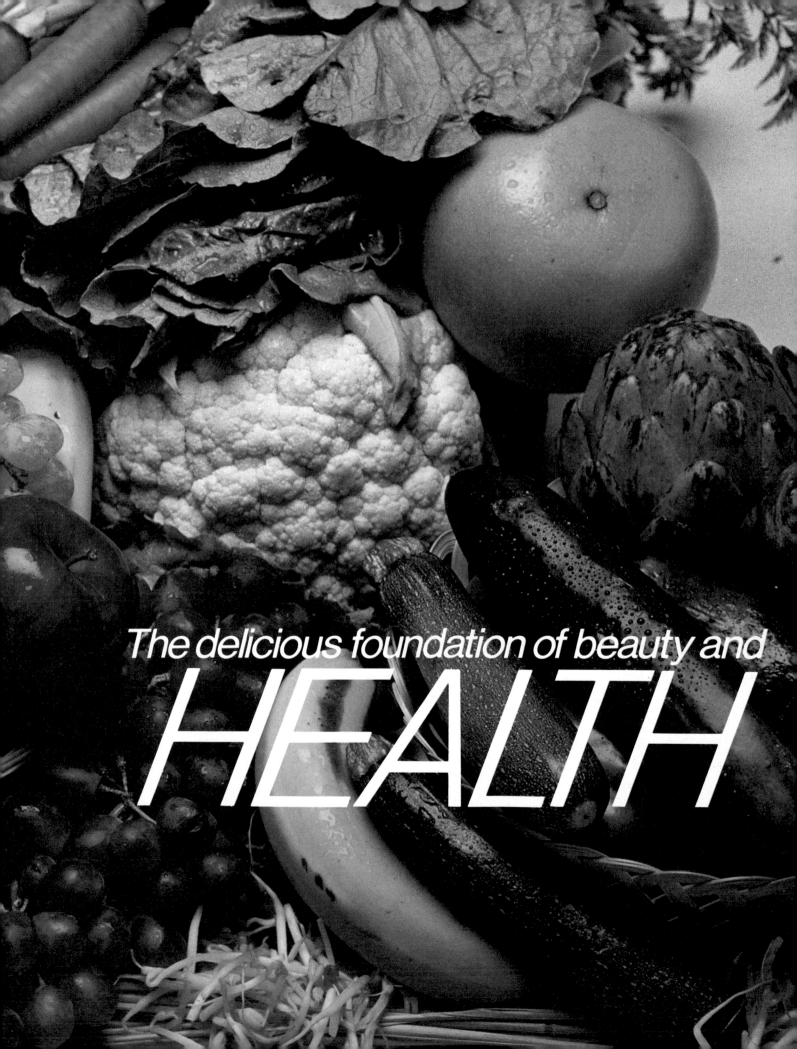

The delicious foundation of beauty and

HEALTH

A new way of eating with health and beauty in mind

Just as glorious hair and a glowing complexion are the rewards of the perfect kind of hair and skin care, vibrant good health is the reward of a carefully thought-out diet. The beauty secret for achieving boundless energy and head-to-toe good looks is as simple as eating delicious and wholesome foods.

Interestingly enough, most women know these beauty foods without being told. Food that looks pretty in its raw state: cold, crisp red apples and golden cereal grains, for instance; plump tomatoes; ruddy ripe peaches; luscious blue-black grapes; all the nutrition-filled bounty that comes from the land will make you pretty, too.

Somehow, too, the really healthful foods almost always seem to taste good together almost any way you combine them. For either a dessert or a snack that everyone enjoys, try a medley of fresh ripe fruits sliced into a crystal bowl, drizzled with honey and sprinkled with fresh orange juice. It doesn't matter what fruits you mix into the bowl— the result is always delightful.

It's also hard to go wrong with combinations of deep green crispy vegetables for a big salad bowl. Try mixing together several varieties of lettuce—pale, icy green Bibb lettuce; silky red-tip leaf lettuce; crisp spears of rich green romaine lettuce; the tangy, deep green frills of chicory. Then snip in a bit of red cabbage, diced onion, pretty circles of sweet green pepper, and toss with a dressing made of fresh lemon juice and safflower oil. It's hard to say whether this salad bowl is a greater treat for the eyes or for the taste buds. It's definitely a beauty booster because it supplies you with lots of vitamin C, iron, and vitamin A.

Although reading about "good nutrition" can be very boring, doing something about improving the quality and the taste of the food you and your family eat every day can be fun; and it is really fairly simple. Think of it as part of a total kitchen make-over. The result will provide a healthier, prettier you as well as a prettier food center for your home. Here are a few tips to improve your appearance from the inside out.

THE GOOD AND BEAUTIFUL FOODS

Prepare your own fresh fruit drinks. This need not be a time-consuming and expensive proposition. Here's a trick that makes frozen orange juice indistinguishable in taste (it's already equal in nutritive value) from fresh-squeezed juice. To a 48-ounce bottle of reconstituted frozen orange juice, add the juice and some of the pulp from 2 freshly squeezed oranges. Stir well. The taste is transformed, and everyone who drinks it will think it is *fresh* juice. Use this fresh orange juice as the basis for a long, cold, fresh orangeade. Pour 2 tablespoons orange juice into a tall glass. Add ice cubes and a wheel of thin-sliced lemon; then fill with bubbling bottled water for a fizzy, refreshing drink that's low in calories. At other times, instead of orange juice, you might substitute a little juice of whatever fruit is fresh. How about a long, cool rosy-pink drink made from fresh strawberries? For each drink, mash a few berries in a strainer. To the juice add a little honey, and fill the glass with sparkling water. Float a whole strawberry in the glass and garnish with a sprig of fresh mint.

Collect a variety of flavors of herbal teas—you can find dozens of these at many supermarkets and at all health-food shops—to enjoy hot or iced. Some of these teas take time to get used to; others are real crowd pleasers. Peppermint tea, chamomile tea, and pink hibiscus-flower tea are three that a great many people enjoy. When iced, they combine beautifully with fruit juices for intriguing, delicious, and healthful long drinks. Try combining spicy, tart rose-hips tea with apple juice for a tangy cold drink, or iced peppermint tea with grape juice for a delicious but definitely mysterious flavor.

A COLORFUL REFRIGERATOR

Fresh healthful drinks can help you create a more attractive refrigerator. Imagine the rainbow effect of a refrigerator filled with covered pitchers and glass jars of fruit juices, ades, and iced teas—especially if you garnish them with wheels of citrus slices, cinnamon sticks, sprigs of fresh mint, or fresh basil (yes, fresh basil; it's a wonderful minty taste with just a tang of difference when used to flavor iced tea). Because fruit juices often settle after standing, and need stirring before you pour, have a natural wooden chopstick on hand for each pitcher of juice. The bamboo adds no metallic flavor, spares your ears the clank of metal spoon against glass, and looks decorative in a natural, practical way. (A package of chopsticks can be bought for under a dollar at an Oriental gift shop or a housewares store, and the chopsticks are reusable.)

You'll also want to have all the ingredients for a platter of *crudités*, the chilly, crisp bites of raw vegetables that satisfy the most gnawing hunger attacks without adding up to an overload of calories. Strips of carrots, raw crunchy string beans, little buds of raw cauliflower, juicy celery sticks—all of these should be right there at hand in the fridge when hunger strikes. Use the blender to whip together a dip of yogurt and chives and lemon juice if you wish, or just enjoy the raw cold vegetables *au naturel*.

Your gorgeous refrigerator can also store the makings of an appetizing, healthy meal that doesn't even require cooking. If you have on hand a container of plain yogurt, a jar of crunchy golden wheat germ, and some fresh fruit, you can put together a beautiful light lunch or snack in a matter of seconds:
Slice or puree a fresh peach or banana in a bowl, spoon creamy plain yogurt over the fruit, sprinkle with wheat germ, stir, and enjoy the various textures and flavors.

You'll get lots of B vitamins, vitamin C, potassium, calcium, and protein.

When shopping, buy only enough fresh fruit and vegetables to satisfy your needs for the next three or four days. If you feel the refrigerator looks bare (it often does if you live alone), buy some extra lemons and oranges (they have great lasting power, are even juicier and just as full of vitamin C when their skins begin to shrivel slightly); get a big bunch of parsley to stand—like flowers—in a glass of water in the refrigerator. It's surprising how cheery and pretty parsley looks. Onions in a wicker basket can also be kept in the refrigerator for a long period.

If you find you have bought too much of any fresh food, plan to use it promptly. Look through your cookbooks for recipes that call for a quantity of the food you have oversupplied. If you have overripe bananas on hand, use them in a quick banana bread. And if you are dieting and shouldn't eat banana bread, make it and take it to a friend or neighbor as a little just-thinking-of-you present. Be on the lookout, too, for household hints that help you store and conserve foods. Here's one for celery that's gone limp in the food crisper: place the celery in a bowl of cold water, store overnight in the refrigerator. Next day the celery will be crunchy again, and it will last another few days.

Eating for beauty and health is enhanced by a handsome, natural setting for food preparation and enjoyment. Natural materials—pretty woven baskets of straw and cane, wood bowls and trays—seem to fit right in and make appealing additions to any kitchen. Put up a few nails and hang some good-looking baskets on your kitchen walls. This can help remind you to use your basket collection. Wouldn't a big basket filled with ripe russet apples look pretty on the kitchen counter? Especially when you consider that eating an apple, raw and unpeeled, works as a natural toothbrush to clean your teeth and help keep them plaque-free. A wooden salad bowl needn't be used only for salads. Think how good your teakwood salad bowl would look piled high with tawny ripe pears, or with walnuts or almonds in their pale golden shells.

But suppose the problem is not one of encouraging yourself and your family to eat in a healthful way, but rather of curbing a tendency to overindulge in the pleasures of the table?

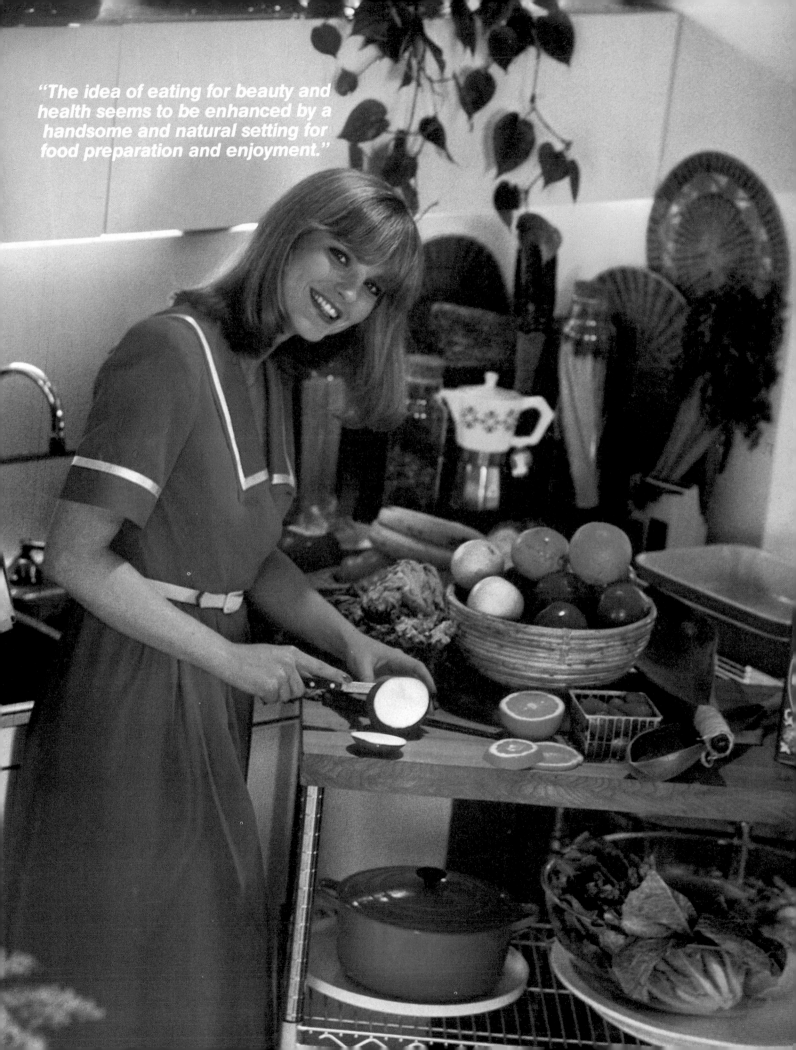

"The idea of eating for beauty and health seems to be enhanced by a handsome and natural setting for food preparation and enjoyment."

The winner's way with weight control

Although it sometimes seems that dieting is the national pastime, 40 percent of all Americans are 20 pounds or more over their ideal weight. Weight-control experts say that only one person in five who set out to lose weight achieves the desired weight goal and maintains it. What is that successful dieter's secret?

The winning dieter is the one who decides on her own whether or not she needs to lose weight and whether or not she really and truly wants to. Going on a diet involves a serious commitment and a willingness to sacrifice. The dieter must be motivated and willing to make a lifelong change for the better both in the kinds and amounts of food she eats and in the attitude she has toward food in general. Then she can face the weight-control problem and develop a habit of eating that will assure her she will never again be plagued by extra pounds and inches. If weight loss is only a temporary fluctuation, part of an unhealthy up-and-down pattern known as the Yo-Yo Syndrome, then all the effort made in going on a diet is eventually wasted. The important aspect of diet is to make it a comfortable part of everyday life.

SHOULD YOU GO ON A DIET?

Only you can answer that.

The chart of desirable weights below can help you get an idea of what you should weigh—to conform to healthful guidelines for your height and frame—but your own eye will tell you more accurately if a diet is in order. Again use your mirror as you have for all the other facets of your beauty analysis. After a bath, study yourself: look at all the angles, all the curves. If you find there's more of you than pleases your eye, then you should diet. Your next decisions involve when and how.

Timing is important for successful dieting. Don't plan to begin a diet just before starting a new job, taking a vacation, or having your mother-in-law come for a visit. These and other occasions that involve change and stress are bad times to add further strain by altering your eating routine and, possibly, the kinds of food you will be eating.

How you trim your caloric intake is extremely important; the diet that works perfectly for your next-door neighbor could be all wrong for you if it is unsuited to your temperament. Before attempting to follow a specific diet, ask yourself how well it fits into your life pattern. Do you demand orderliness and predictability for happiness? Or does that smack of monotony and drab routine to you? Your answer can help you decide on a diet. If you thrive on change and variety, don't choose a diet that requires you to adhere to the same menu day after day or to a certain food that must be eaten at every meal. Your eventual response will be to kick over the traces and run away from your regimen.

If you are the sort of person who dislikes change, you are apt to be most comfortable if your new weight-loss diet is planned around familiar foods, even though these may now be prepared differently and you will be eating smaller quantities of them.

desirable weights for women age 25 and over

(WEIGHT IN POUNDS ACCORDING TO FRAME)

HEIGHT FEET	HEIGHT INCHES	SMALL FRAME	MEDIUM FRAME	LARGE FRAME
4	10	92–98	96–107	104–119
4	11	94–101	98–110	106–122
5	0	96–104	101–113	109–125
5	1	99–107	104–116	112–128
5	2	102–110	107–119	115–131
5	3	105–113	110–122	118–134
5	4	108–116	113–126	121–138
5	5	111–119	116–130	125–142
5	6	114–123	120–135	129–146
5	7	118–127	124–139	133–150
5	8	122–131	128–143	137–154
5	9	126–135	132–147	141–158
5	10	130–140	136–151	145–163
5	11	134–144	140–155	149–168
6	0	138–148	144–159	153–173

Metropolitan Life Insurance Company

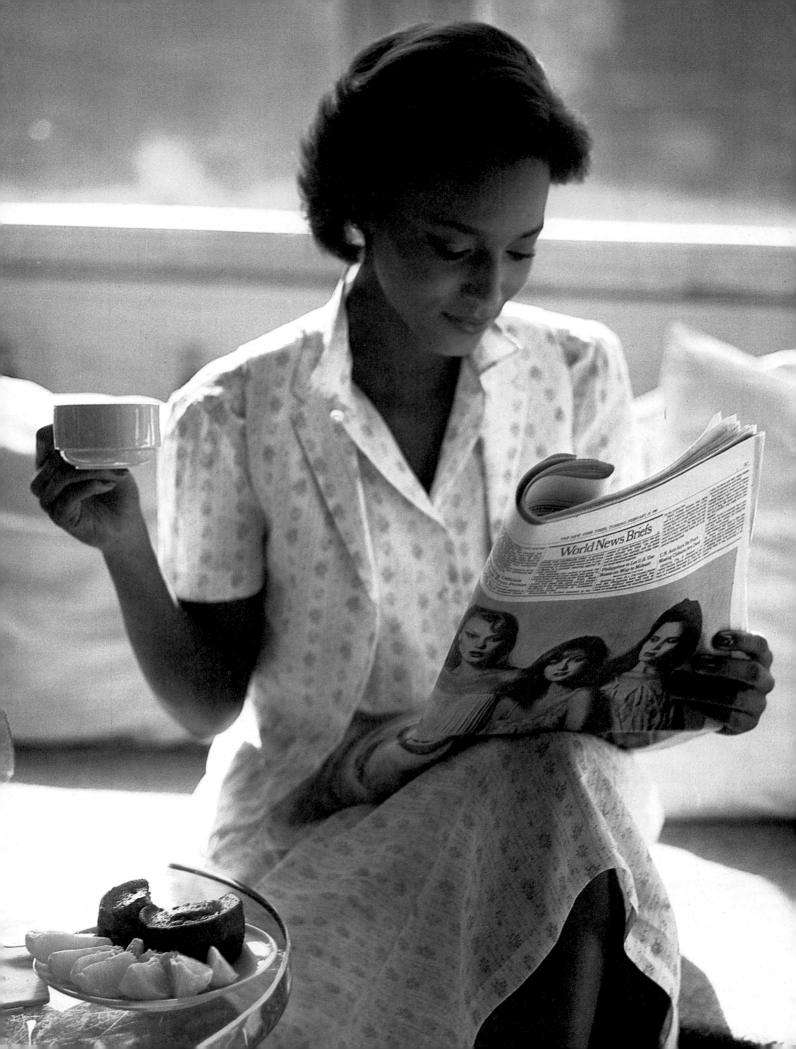

USE YOUR BEAUTY NOTEBOOK

In order to understand your own individual pattern of overeating, as well as to facilitate choosing the diet plan that will be most comfortable for you to follow, it's a good idea to begin by keeping a diet diary for one week. Use your spiral-bound beauty notebook. Keep it in your handbag at all times, and every time you eat or drink anything—one cookie or an entire meal—write it down. Make five headings across the top of the page: When . . . What . . . Where . . . Who . . . Why. Draw lines down the page to make five columns. Then, with each snack or meal, make the appropriate entries. The time of day, what you ate, where you were when you ate it, who was with you, and how you felt at the time (bored, lonely, angry . . .).

Keep a diet diary for a week and you will be surprised to discover your own secrets. You will probably find that by keeping a diary, you can keep your weight down without calorie counting. Knowing that you have to get out your notebook and write it down will help you avoid having a bite here and there during the day. More important, the diary will cause you to become aware of your patterns of hunger, and of the "sneak eating" that can be a dieter's downfall—finishing off something the kids didn't eat, or absentmindedly tasting as you prepare meals. You'll also learn to be aware of the temptation to eat out of boredom. It's a common response.

No matter what diet plan you choose, don't skip breakfast. It's the meal that sets the tone of the day.

Especially when dieting you need the energy that breakfast provides. Breakfast also strengthens your will to resist diet-destroying snacks in the hours before lunch.

Many people who skip breakfast do so because preparation would take too much time. One way around that is to fix breakfast the night before. Or prepare breakfast for the whole week on one evening. Delicious foods that you can make ahead include egg custards and bran muffins.

Each morning you can eat a healthy, hearty breakfast without rushing. After a good breakfast, look in the refrigerator and the cabinets to make your selections for the food you will eat that day. Planning the day's food in advance helps you avoid overeating and impulsive, reckless food choices made when you are hungry. Menu planning—using only what is at hand—is designed to eliminate the temptation to buy food you don't need, a classic pitfall of shopping when you're hungry.

One important thing to remember is that even the woman who is properly motivated, who selects her time and makes her plan for dieting carefully, can slip off her diet. It isn't the end of the world, nor should it spell the end of your resolve to lose weight.

Don't write off your diet as a failure (or, worse, yourself as weak-willed and worthless) because you succumb to a forbidden high-calorie treat or even to a whole weekend of reckless indulgence. Don't feel guilty. Just get back as quickly as you can to the healthful new diet routine you have begun.

"No matter what diet plan you choose, don't skip breakfast. It's the meal that sets the tone for the day."

IT'S ALL A QUESTION OF CALORIES

In choosing a diet, you cannot avoid the fact that calorie requirements are quite specific. Body weight and the degree of energy output determine the precise amount of food your body needs.

Simple arithmetic will show you how many calories are needed to maintain your weight and meet your body's energy requirements.

Multiply your weight by 15. If you are normally active, the figure you arrive at is the number of calories you need each day to maintain your current weight. As an example, say you weigh 125 pounds: $125 \times 15 = 1,875$ calories to maintain it.

If you are very active, you can eat more without gaining weight. In fact, you need more food in order to maintain your weight. If you run and jog each day, swim, play tennis, or keep active in some other way for a weekly total of five to six hours, add 200 to the figure. So, $1,875 + 200 = 2,075$ calories it takes to maintain your proper weight.

If you seldom or never engage in sports or vigorous exercise, subtract 200. Thus, $1,875 - 200 = 1,675$ calories per day in order to avoid gaining weight.

If the body is supplied with more calories than it needs, it will store the excess as fat reserves against future need. Should a time arrive when the body gets less than the daily total it demands, it will signal with hunger; then, should the calories not be forthcoming, it will begin to draw upon the stockpile of fat reserves, using this source for its needs. This is when you begin to lose weight. But this happens slowly. Each pound of body weight represents a total of 3,500 calories oversupplied in the past. To lose weight, the body must be coaxed into spending that calorie reserve.

Providing the body with no calories at all should do the trick . . . in theory only. In fact, unsupervised fasting is dangerous. You lose weight on a fast, but too quickly for the skin to recontour itself, so that you will be left with a drawn, haggard look that's more sick than svelte, plus skin that sags like an outsize leotard.

The only safe and becoming way to lose weight is the slow and steady way. Subtract 600 calories from your present daily intake in order to lose a pound a week. For two pounds a week, cut back 1,200 calories each day. A loss of two pounds each week is the most you should aim for in a good weight-reduction program. And don't eat less than 1,200 calories a day unless specifically instructed to do so by your doctor.

A calorie is a calorie. The body doesn't know whether it comes from a steak or a cupcake. And it doesn't care, as long as the calorie can be metabolized for energy. But where you get your calories does affect the state of your health, so get them from the most wholesome sources.

The chart below can be used to plan an ideal dieting pattern to suit your individual requirements. If you are happier having three balanced meals a day, eat three meals. If you are a "snacker," always tempted to eat between meals, plan a series of 6 mini-meals spaced throughout the day, but using a reduced quantity of food at each "meal."

BASIC INGREDIENTS OF A BALANCED 1,200-CALORIE DAILY DIET PLAN

1 pint (2 cups) skim milk

1 egg (limit eggs to two or three a week)

5 ounces lean meat, poultry, liver, fish, or cheese

½ cup whole-grain cereal

1 small potato

3 slices whole-grain bread

1 serving green or yellow vegetables (raw, steamed, or microwave-prepared, without sauce)

2 servings of other vegetables

1 citrus fruit

1 tomato or glass of tomato juice

2 servings of other fruit (fresh raw, or unsweetened if canned or frozen)

3 teaspoons margarine or polyunsaturated liquid vegetable oil

FOR OPTIMUM HEALTH, WHATEVER YOUR CALORIE TOTAL:

Plan to get more fiber in your diet through eating fresh raw fruits and vegetables as often as possible. Try to cut back on refined carbohydrates, such as white flour, white sugar, and the cakes and pastries made from them. Cut back on fat, especially saturated animal fats, and keep your salt intake as low as your doctor considers wise. Alcohol is very high in calories and not nourishing; its consumption should be limited.

If you are the sort of person who must have a no-choice diet, there are many books available to plan your program. But if you need no rigid plan, just make sure you keep your calorie intake to 1,200 per day from a wide variety of wholesome foods that will enhance your health naturally.

DEALING WITH THE URGE TO CHEAT ON YOUR DIET

There are times when even the best little dieter in the world feels an almost uncontrollable urge to feast, to overindulge in food. It's an absolutely normal response to a period of careful, self-limiting behavior.

There is a way to indulge in a little binge eating without wrecking your diet. Instead of satisfying the sudden urge for rich sweets, have a bunch of grapes (65 calories in 8 ounces).

Below are some other suggestions for healthful low-calorie snacking.

FOOD	QUANTITY	CALORIES
Artichoke with lemon	1 whole	55
Artichoke heart with lemon	1 heart	5
Breadsticks	1	10
Cauliflower, raw	1 cup	24
Dill pickle	1 large	10
Honeydew melon balls	1 cup	50
Jellied madrilene soup	1 cup	45
Mushrooms, fresh raw sliced	1 cup	20
Oyster crackers	1	3
Popcorn, light salt, no butter	1 cup	25
Watermelon balls	1 cup	25

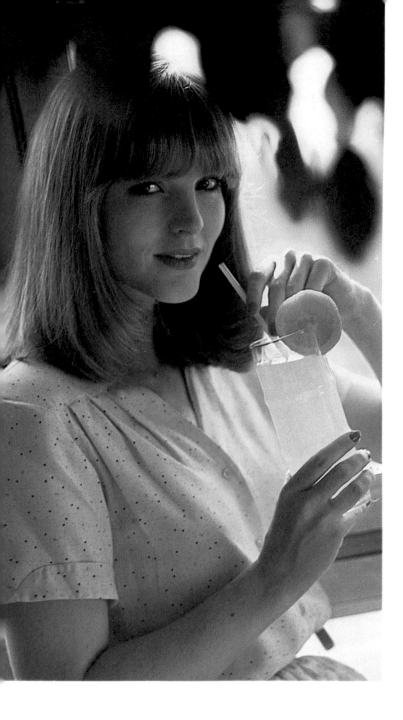

A LIST OF 20 TIPS AND SUGGESTIONS TO HELP YOU BECOME A SUCCESSFUL DIETER

1. Never skip meals. That leads to fatigue, to irritability, and often to late-night binging.

2. Always sit down at a table when you eat, whether a full meal or a quick snack. It's easy to "just pick" a surprising number of calories standing and eating from the kitchen cupboard or the refrigerator. Making the effort to take food to the table causes you to become more aware of what you are eating and how much.

3. Never take a second bite of food until you've swallowed the first. Put down your fork, chew thoroughly, then swallow. You'll aid digestion, and eating slowly leads to eating less. Feelings of hunger do not subside until the level of blood sugar rises, and it takes almost twenty minutes for the food you eat to produce this elevation of the blood-sugar level. If you bolt down your food, you are apt to overeat.

4. Small portions look much bigger when served on smaller plates. Use a luncheon-size instead of the dinner-size plate, or have your dinner on a salad plate.

5. Make the meal a treat for your senses. Be especially concerned, when dieting, to make meals attractive. A low-calorie dinner can be a high-style occasion. How about candles and real linen napkins? Or lay in a store of inexpensive, beautifully designed paper place mats, napkins and coated paper plates in a variety of pretty colors and patterns. You'll spend less on a week's worth of festive colors for the table than you would on just one diet-wrecking cake from the bakery.

6. If you have children, make the start of a diet the start of Mother's Lib. Let them fix their own snacks, and you won't be tempted to have a bite of peanut butter or whatever.

7. If your problem isn't eating between meals but overeating at meals (your diary will tell you within a week), then treat yourself to an extra course shortly before mealtime. Have a filling, but low-calorie, treat fifteen minutes before dinner and you'll be less inclined to overeat. Icy cold raw vegetable sticks are good. Try cucumber slivers, carrot sticks, flowerettes of cauliflower, kept chilled and ready.

8. A hot drink can conquer hunger pangs between meals, yet add practically no calories. Try a hot herbal tea blend, or a cup of vegetable bouillon.

9. Learn your snack signals. If you always make a trip to the refrigerator or the office snack bar at 3 P.M., then choose that exact time to brush your hair and freshen your makeup instead. Break out of your rut.

10. Substitutions, low-calorie for high-calorie, are the salvation for anyone who enjoys eating but has to watch calories. But when you're saving a calorie here, a few calories there, it's hard to see the big picture and realize just how big a difference the small substitutions make. It seems a winning, worthwhile game if you keep track with a list. With every low-calorie substitution, note the calories saved. Smaller portions save calories too; when you cut back from a bigger piece to a smaller, jot down the calorie difference. Total your calories saved at the end of the day. You'll be pleased and surprised.

11. Serve plates in the kitchen, directly from the stove; then take only the food that is on your plate to the table. No serving bowls full of food means less dishwashing and discourages diet-defeating second helpings.

12. Leftovers are the bane of a dieter's existence. If you can't bear to throw food away, and polish off the last little bits of a dish just to "get it out of the way," start to reorganize your cooking to save your diet. Plot meals carefully so you don't cook more food than needed. If you realize you have prepared too much of a dish, think about freezing part for another meal. (Many foods, however, freeze better and retain more nutrients if frozen before cooking.) When there are leftovers, refrigerate them promptly and plan to make them the basis of tomorrow's meal, not the ruination of today's diet.

13. Have supportive people around you at meals whenever possible. Eating alone leads to overeating for many of us. How about making plans for a regular, standing lunch date with a couple of friends who are also watching the scale? You can discuss your diets and your progress with them at these lunches, trade tips and ideas, and swap your own experiences in living well without overeating.

14. Give yourself little nonfood rewards for sticking to the new eating plan. Add up the money you *didn't* spend on dessert, or a pastry with your coffee break, and buy yourself a lipstick in a terrific new shade at the end of the week. Or put a quarter aside for each day you stay within your calorie limit, and buy yourself a weekly treat.

15. Make weight loss less abstract, more real. If you want to lose 10 pounds, it helps to know what 10 pounds feels like. In the supermarket, pick up two 5-pound bags of flour and walk a little way down the aisle with them. When you replace the bags on the shelf, see how much better you feel without that burden. Imagine how much better you're going to feel after shedding the equal burden you carry around all the time when you are overweight.

16. Set a goal for yourself. You might buy a new dress in the smaller size you plan to wear, or a new body-hugging swimsuit. Looking forward to being able to wear this will help keep your mind on the rewards of a diet.

17. Don't make telephone calls from the kitchen, if possible. A cozy chat with a friend, or an upsetting one with the TV repairman, can trigger the urge to eat. It will pass, but not if you're standing at the refrigerator. If you must use the telephone in the kitchen, keep your hands busy. Wipe the countertop, polish silver—just don't eat.

18. Keep some kind of busywork for your hands beside the chair where you watch television. Even if other members of the family snack while they watch, you can resist if you're doing some productive knitting.

19. When you go out with friends to a restaurant for dinner, make a low-calorie selection that suits your diet and say "no" politely to any and all invitations to sample "just a bite" of what your companions ordered. It may be delicious, but you'll regret it later.

20. Overcome the habit of eating when you're bored. Don't get bored. Instead of sitting there nibbling because you have nothing to do, get up and go out for a short walk or a run. Go out to a museum or a movie if there's lots of time; if not, spend a little time on your hands: touch up your manicure with another coat of enamel, or just massage some cuticle cream around the base of your nails. Get busy. It will help you get slim.

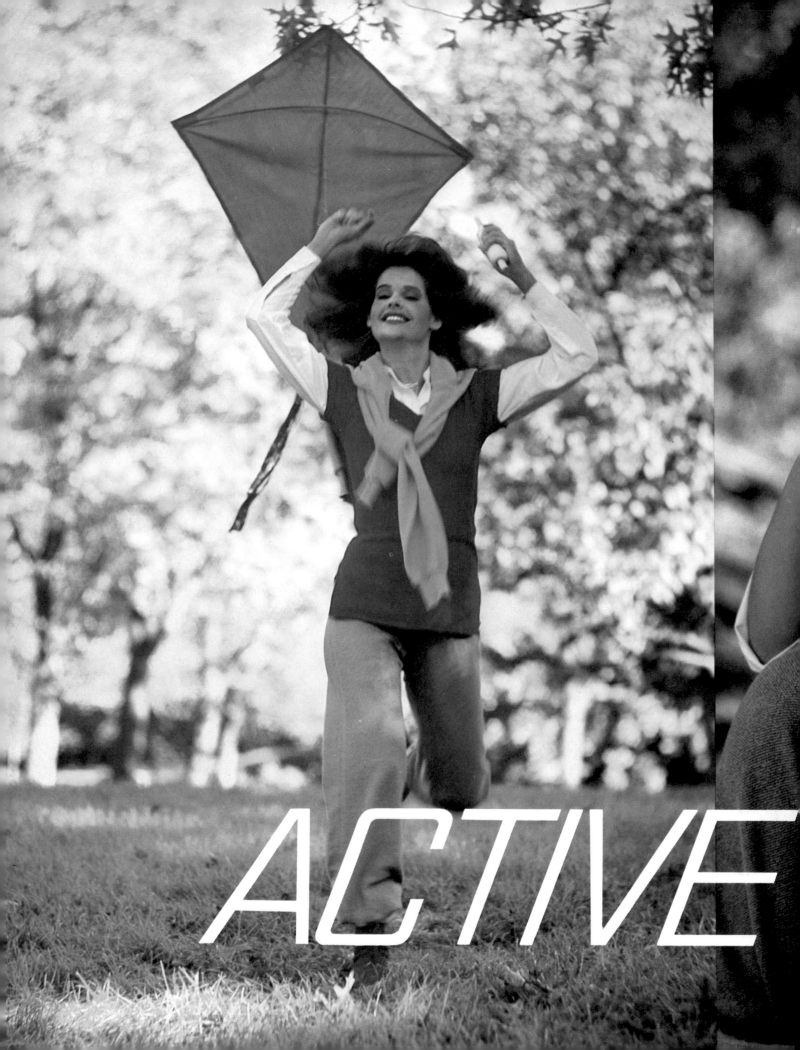

ACTIVE

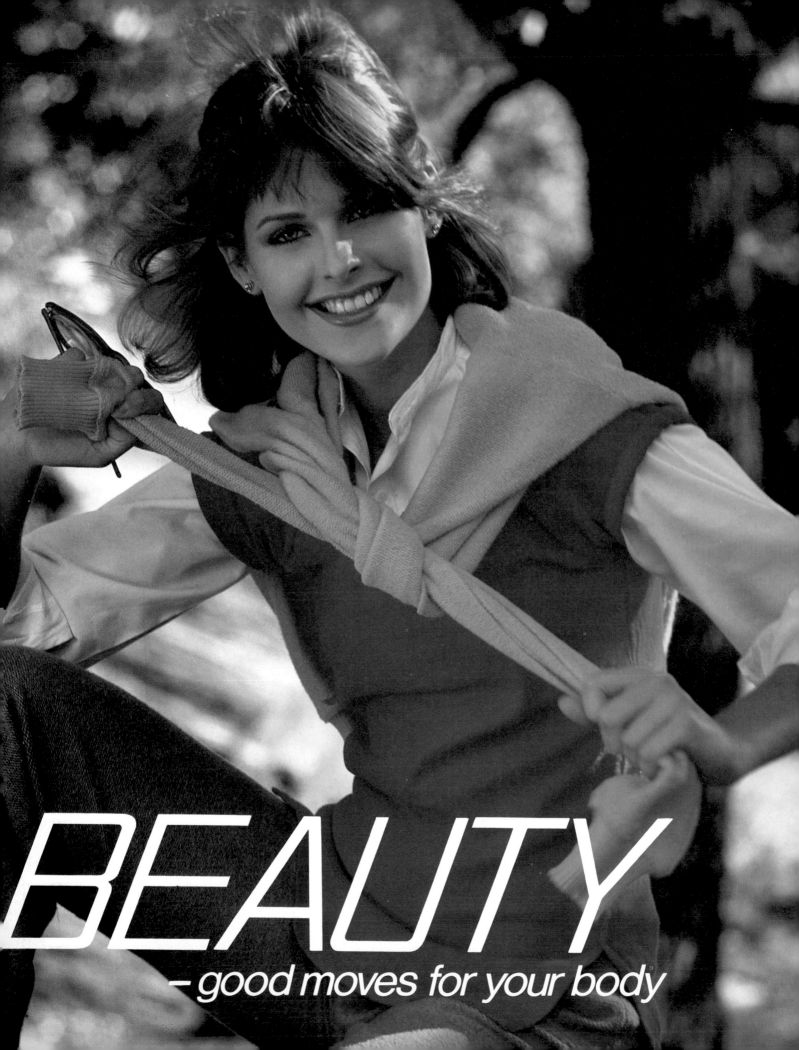

BEAUTY
– good moves for your body

Play your way to fitness

All the good things you do for yourself are better and more effective if you let your body become more active. With just a little increase in your exercise schedule, your circulation will step up; and an increase in circulation provides more beautiful skin, hair, and stronger nails.

You needn't devote your life to exercise (although some very sportive people might find the idea appealing). In less than thirty minutes a day you can have a firmer, shapelier body by following one or a combination of the three programs given here. But before starting any new exercise program, have your doctor give you a thorough checkup to confirm that your intended program is safe for you.

Perhaps you feel that even an extra thirty minutes is hard to come by in your crowded daily schedule. Consider the early morning as a possibility. Even if you are the sort of woman who "just can't function until noon," you may be surprised to find that getting up while the world is still sleeping and going out for a run to greet the day actually helps you get through a long, busy day with serenity. Many, many women wouldn't miss that early-morning run on nice days, or that early session of rope skipping indoors during poor weather. They claim there is a very soothing and aesthetically satisfying quality about savoring the stillness of the early hours as you begin to put your body into motion for the day.

If the morning is really not possible, or if end-of-the-day exercise is better for psychological or practical reasons, then try to make that half hour an essential gift to yourself. Shedding the day's accumulation of tensions and concerns during a good session of huff-and-puff physical activity is a perfect antidote for a woman who spends all day in an office or at housework. It can be a start for a "second day," and exercise at the close of the day ensures that you will be relaxed and glowing as you begin the activities of the evening.

Then again, you might find that a midday exercise break suits you best. Any time of the day that is convenient and comfortable is a good time for becoming more active. But do make it a regular part of your schedule. Consider this an important appointment with yourself, an unbreakable date—like your once-a-week Beauty Time—for you to get in touch with your own body. Just as in every other area of beauty care, study yourself in the mirror to know the current state of your looks. Every exercise date with yourself, if kept, will be reflected by a more perfect image.

Use the mirror, too, to check your position and your progress if you are doing specific indoor exercises. Do your exercises before a full-length mirror when possible: it helps develop grace of movement. Being able to actually *see* the muscles of your body at work can help inspire you to stick to it, whatever your exercise routine.

The simplest, easiest exercise—even for the woman who is resolutely anti-exercise—is a limbering stretch in the morning. This not only helps you feel better, it starts you moving more gracefully each day.

A LIMBERING STRETCH
TO AWAKEN THE BODY

■ Stand with legs comfortably apart. Swing arms up and clasp hands over your head. Keeping arms straight, stretch as far to the left as you can. Keep the upper body straight, bending from the waist. Then stretch as far as possible to the right. Do 10 times, 5 times each way.

■ Stand with feet comfortably apart and legs straight. Stretch arms straight out. Bend forward from the waist. Try to let your trunk hang from the hips, with chest and head hanging close in to your legs and arms dangling. Try to touch your right hand to your left foot. Raise your left arm up behind you to help your balance. Return to starting position and reverse the reach, left hand to right foot. Do up to 10 each side.

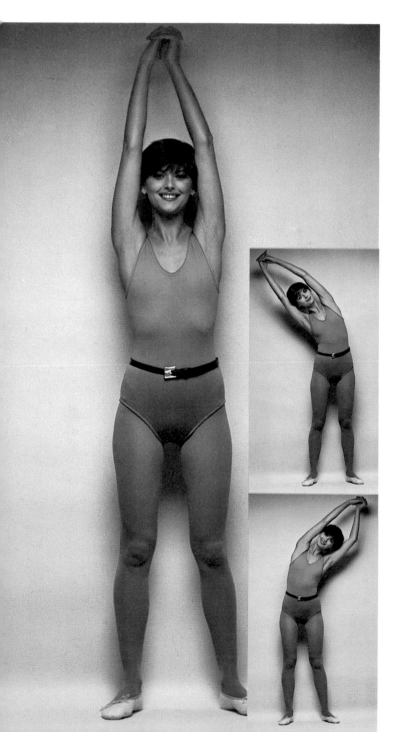

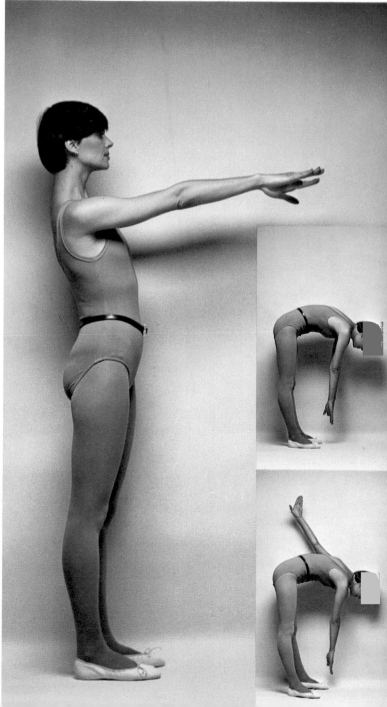

■ Stand with hands placed on your shoulders. Without moving your hands from your shoulders, pretend that you are drawing big *O*s in the air with your elbows. Try to make the circles meet in front of you by bringing your elbows as close together as you can in front as you describe wide circles. Do 5 times.

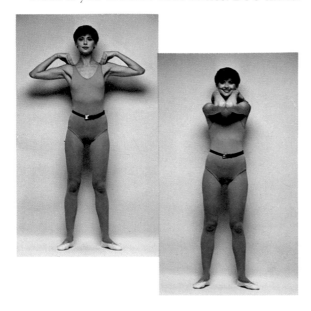

■ Stand with hands clasped behind your back. Keep your back and neck straight and bend from the hips to gradually lower your trunk as if you wanted to touch your forehead to the floor. Go down as far as you can, and feel your hamstring muscles stretching. As you lower your torso, raise your arms, with hands still clasped, for balance. Do 10 times.

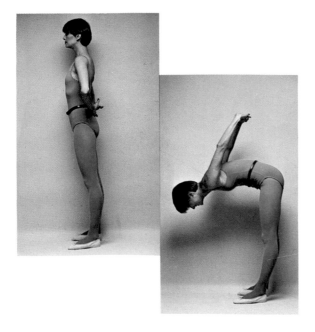

■ Stand and lift your left knee as high as you can, bringing it in close to your chest. Clasp the knee with your hands; then release and lower your leg. Lift and clasp your right knee. Alternate legs almost as if you were running in place. Do up to 10 each side.

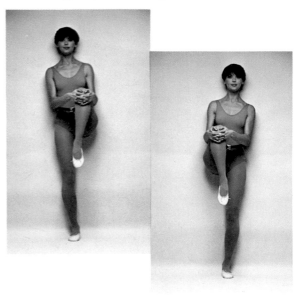

This limbering stretch helps to act as a warm-up for the body before more prolonged exercise such as running or skipping rope. It is also a wonderful relaxer, and you might want to try it before a bath as a further aid to looking and feeling your best.

If you have been inactive lately, you might be tempted to rush into a very ambitious exercise program to make up for lost time. Don't. If your body has been unused to exercise, the gentle series of stretches above will provide quite enough stimulation for the first day. The best way to ease into a more active way of life is to do it by degrees. Begin with a plan that adds movement to your day in easy stages which do not fatigue you but rather make you eager for more.

Let's suppose you have done no exercise in years but your doctor agrees exercise is in order for you. On the first day of your new regimen, take a walk in the fresh air either first thing in the morning or at the end of the day. Walk briskly to the corner of the block, or to the fourth house down the street; then turn around and go back home. Tomorrow, walk to the corner of the next block down the street before retracing your steps. Add just one block to each day's walk. Soon you will find that your little walk covers a surprising distance. Try to increase your speed just a little bit every day, too. Within a couple of weeks you'll be walking a brisk half hour without panting, without tiring; and you will have the benefit of good circulation and a rosy complexion.

As you step up the speed of your walking in the fresh air, it may come to seem more natural to break into a run. The more adventurous may prefer to run a mile rather than walking it. But running is a little more than simply fast walking. It's great for you, but you should do it the right way. Although you can walk in almost any kind of shoe, running demands good running shoes. They needn't be the most expensive "name" brand, but they should fit and support your feet so well that you find them just about your most comfortable shoes. Shop for a pair with a good wide base at the heel, an arch support that is correctly positioned for your foot, and plenty of shock-absorbing cushioning for the entire foot. While good running shoes are essential, a good-looking warm-up suit is not. You can wear anything loose and comfortable to run in. But the chances are that once you wear a warm-up suit, and discover how really comfortable and convenient it is to wear, you'll look forward to a run as an occasion for putting it on.

Choose a course that will be an attractive spot in which to run. The best way to measure the distance is to get into the car and drive to the prettiest, quietest, and safest stretch of the road that's near your house. Use a special tree, or that handsome shingled house, as a landmark. Note the mileage on your car's odometer and drive exactly one-half mile farther. Note another landmark, perhaps a big rhododendron. When you run from the shingled house to the rhododendron and back, you will know that you've run a mile. Until you get into really good shape, you might find that even half a mile is too long for a sustained run. Don't exhaust yourself. Instead, slow from a run to a walk to recover your breath, but go the distance, whether walking or running. And don't be discouraged. Keep on running—every morning or three times a week, but keep at it on a regular basis. The more often you run, the sooner running becomes easy and joyful.

There are days when you simply cannot get out for a run. It's not healthy to run on days when the temperature and humidity both are very high. It's bad for you to run on days when the air is very polluted. And of course, you may not want to go out in a raging storm. On foul-weather days, try jumping rope or running in place in your bedroom, down in the cellar, in the garage, or wherever you can jump without disturbing other people. These exercises will not only keep you fit and trim, they also have a beneficial effect on your cardiovascular system.

You might enjoy adding other little minutes of stepped-up activity here and there throughout the day. If you drive to work, try shaving off a little of the driving distance by parking your car an extra block or so away from work and walking the extra distance. Or if you take a bus, you might get off one short stop before your destination and walk a block or two. Every little bit of activity helps get your body and mind in beautiful, healthy shape.

A fourth program you might adopt is the only one that is definitely an on-and-off affair: spot reducing. Spot exercises are terrific when you are eager to get in great shape for a special occasion—maybe the one that calls for that clinging, figure-revealing dress. As a steady diet, though, spot exercises are just too boring for most people to keep up on a daily basis. With a regular program of exercise, your body will be looking much firmer within the first month. But to help speed things along, these specific spot exercises can correct some common figure problems by toning specific muscle groups. You'll find at least two exercises each for the main spots where bulge and sag most often strike—such as the throat and chin, where jowls, loose-hanging skin, and doubled chins are the enemy. You can actually lift your bosom for a younger, better-looking figure by strengthening the pectoral muscles which underlie your breasts, even though there are, of course, no muscles to exercise in the breasts themselves. Toning and firming the upper arms can appear to take years off your figure and enable you to wear those sleeveless dresses more confidently. And of course, the disadvantages of bulges from the middle down to the knees are painfully obvious and all too easily come by. Running will help trim the measurements of your waist, hips, buttocks, and thighs, but spot exercises are a splendid complement.

In doing these, or any other exercises, concentrate mentally on the muscles that are working; think about the part of your body you are exercising. You actually slim more efficiently when you perform an action with conscious attention to the movement and the results.

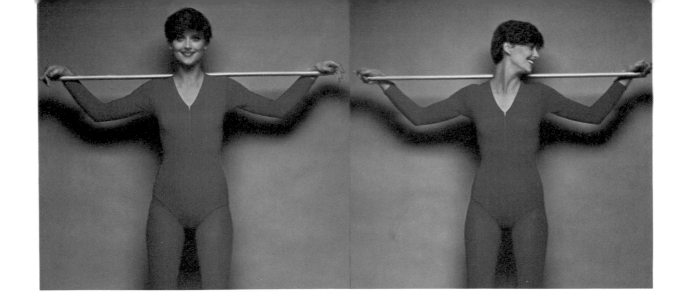

FOR THE THROAT AND CHIN

Hold a broomstick on your shoulders at the back of the neck, your hands grasping the stick near the ends. Turn your head left to right, trying to touch your chin to the stick. Do this 15 times; then reverse, turning your head right to left.

Lie on your back with head hanging over the edge of the bed. Exhale and raise your head toward your chest. Drop your head back, inhaling as you lower your head. Do this 12 times.

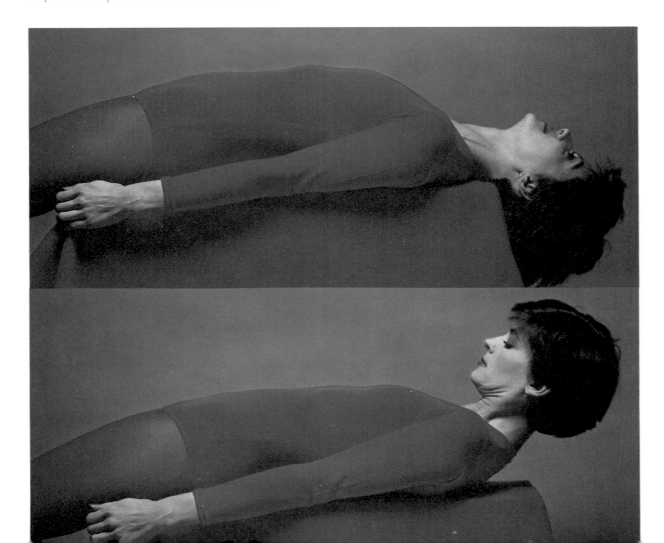

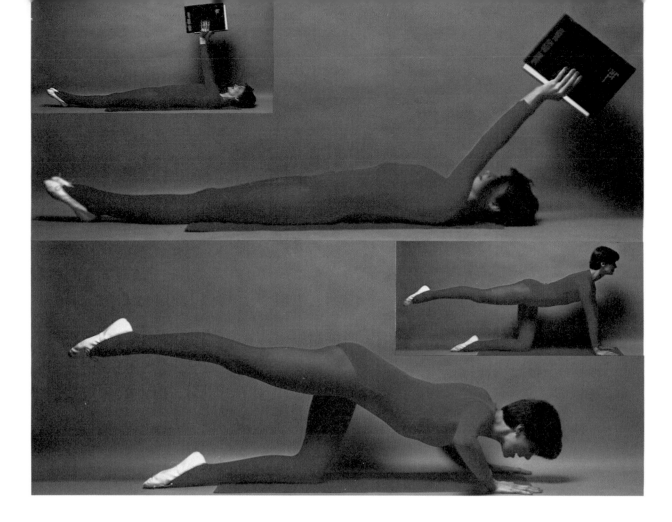

FOR THE BOSOM

Lie on your back on the floor. Hold a 2- to 5-pound weight or a heavy book in each hand with arms straight up and perpendicular to the floor. Slowly lower straight arms to the floor above your head and then to your sides. Start with a few and build up to 10 times each direction.

Get on your hands and knees on an exercise mat or carpeted floor, lift and extend one leg straight from your body. Lower your chest to the floor, keeping leg extended, then raise chest, straightening arms. Do 3 times. Switch legs. Repeat.

Lie on your back and hold your arms straight up; now cross them back and forth above your head in a fast zigzag motion, 12 times.

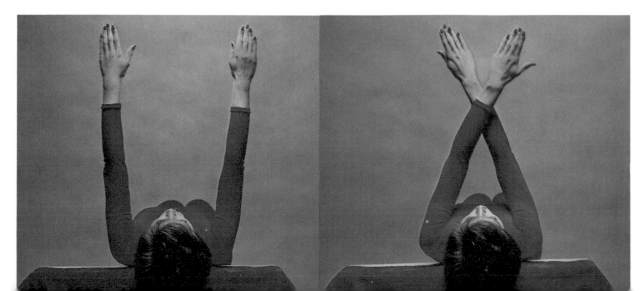

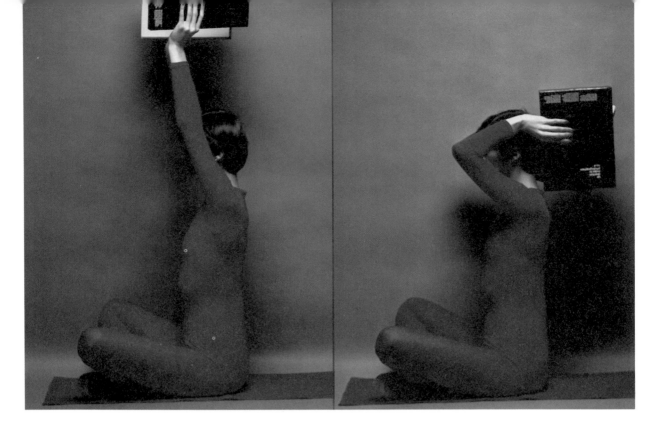

FOR UPPER ARMS

Sit on a bench or a straight chair. Rest your palms flat on the bench, arms straight and fingers pointed forward. Lift your buttocks and thighs off the bench, raise your feet off the floor. Hold for a slow count of 6; relax for a slow count of 3. Do this 6 times.

Sit on the floor or on a chair with your back straight. Hold a 2- to 5-pound weight or a heavy book with both hands up over your head. Slowly bend your arms back and up again. Do this 10 times, keeping your upper arms beside your ears throughout.

Sit on the floor. Grasp a broomstick behind your back with your palms up and hands close together. Push the stick up and down 30 times.

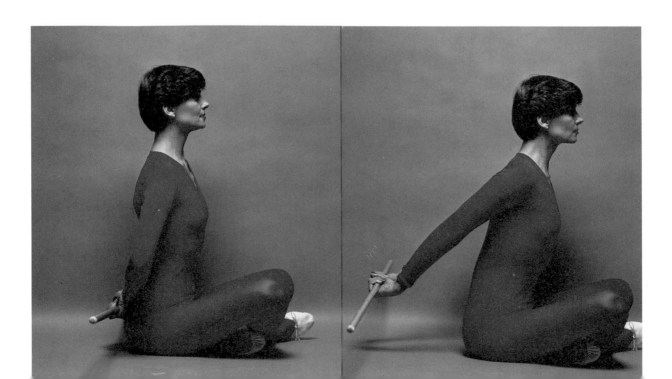

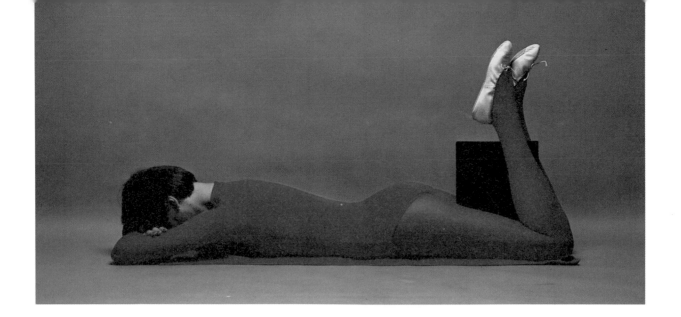

FOR BUTTOCKS

Lie on your stomach on an exercise mat, carpeted floor, or bed. Place a book between your lower thighs and squeeze the book with your thighs. Flex your knees and lift them. Hold for a slow count of 6; relax for a slow count of 3. Do this 6 times.

Stand with your hands clasped at one end of a broomstick, with the other end resting on the floor. Swing your leg forward and back as far as possible. Alternate left and right legs. Do 30 times each.

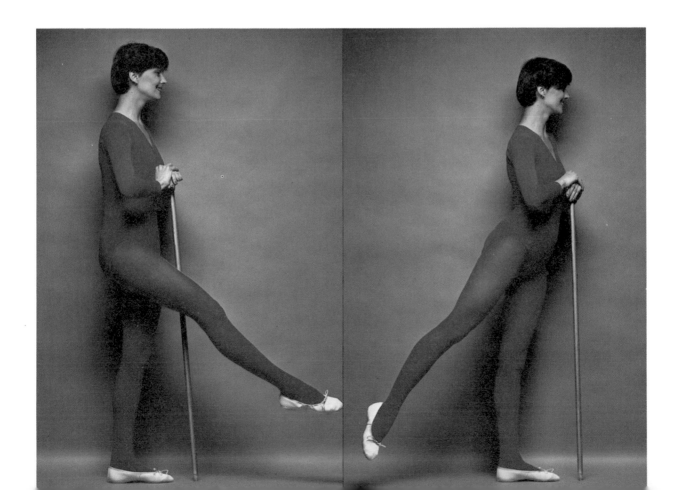

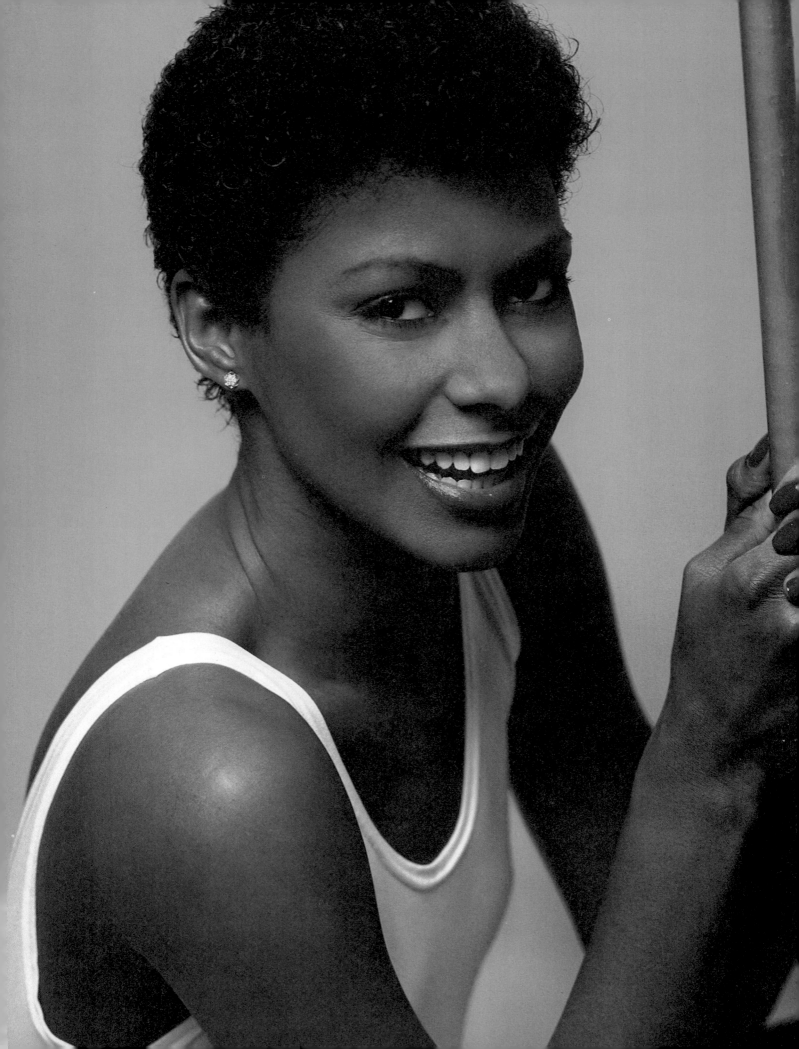

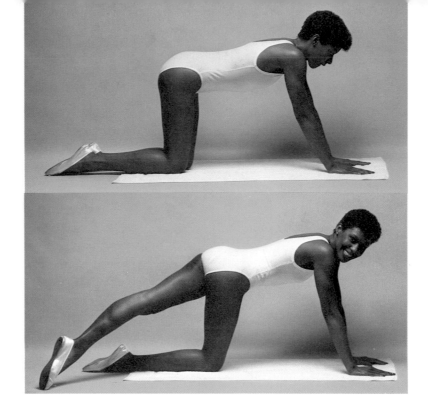

FOR HIPS

Kneel on all fours on the floor, arms straight, elbows locked. Straighten your right leg and swing it over to the left side and back again without touching your foot to the floor. Do 6 times, then reverse, swinging your left leg to the right 6 times.

Sit on a carpeted floor or exercise mat. Sit on your right buttock with your knees flexed to the right side. Hold a broomstick with a wide grip. Swing the stick to the left. Keep your weight to the left side until the left buttock touches the floor as arms swing right. Alternate sides and do 12 times each side.

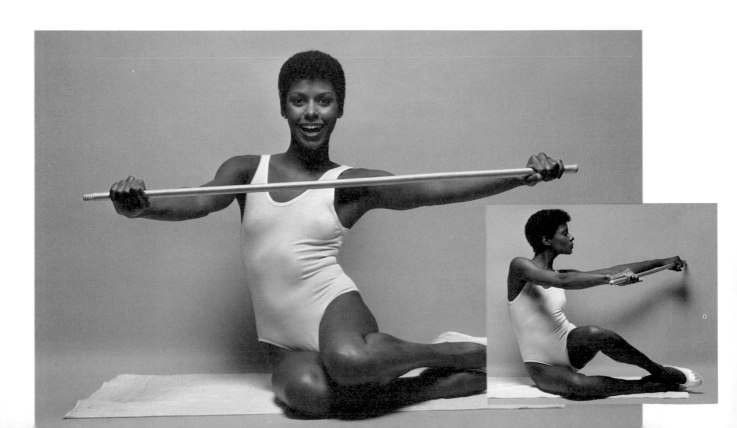

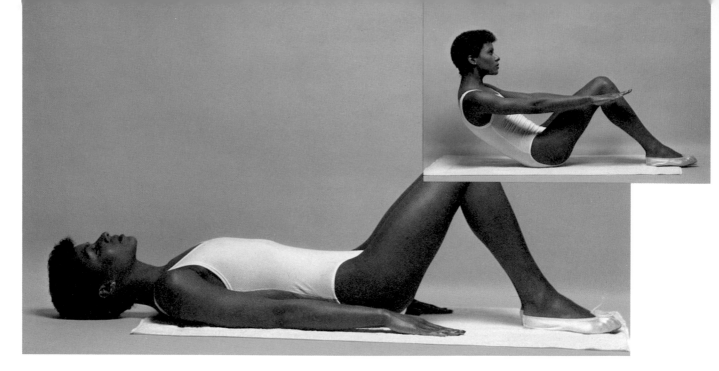

FOR ABDOMEN

Lie on an exercise mat or carpeted floor, knees bent, feet flat on floor and arms out toward your knees. Slowly roll your body up, stretching your fingertips toward the knees. Round the back and tense the abdominal muscles by pulling in the abdomen and exhale while raising the body. Hold the raised position for a slow count of 6. Lower your body slowly, inhaling as you return to the floor. Relax for a count of 3. Do this 6 times.

Sit on the floor. Grasp a broomstick near the ends with both hands. Draw knees up. Hold the stick out in front of your knees; move your legs over the stick as if jumping rope. Do 10 times.

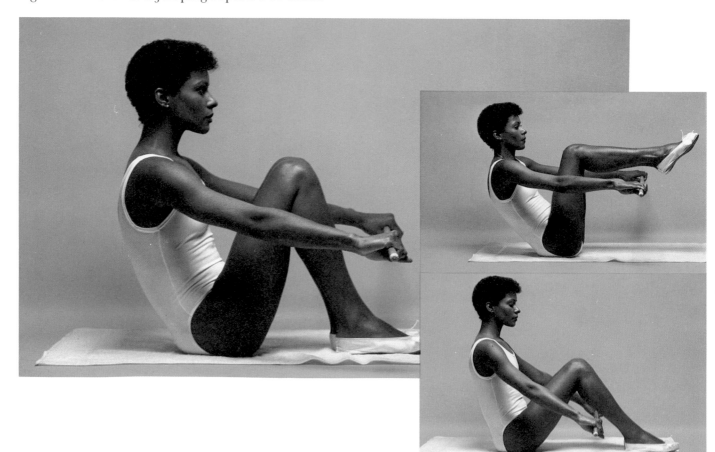

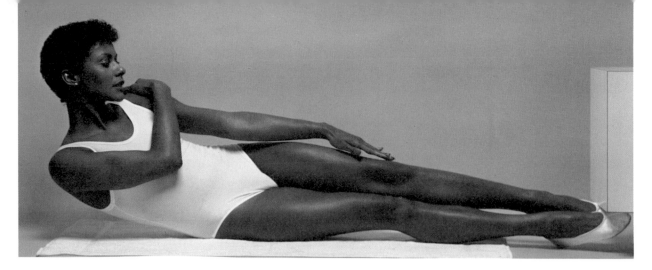

FOR WAISTLINE

Lie on a carpeted floor on your right side with both feet under the edge of a bed or a sofa heavy enough to serve as an anchor. Grasp your left shoulder with your right hand. Rise sideways and reach for your knee with the left hand. Hold for a slow count of 6; relax for a slow count of 6. Reverse. Do this 6 times for each side.

Stand with feet comfortably apart. Hold a broomstick on your shoulders at the back of your neck with arms outstretched and hands resting on the stick near the ends. Bend from side to side, up and down; then twist from side to side. Do 30 times.

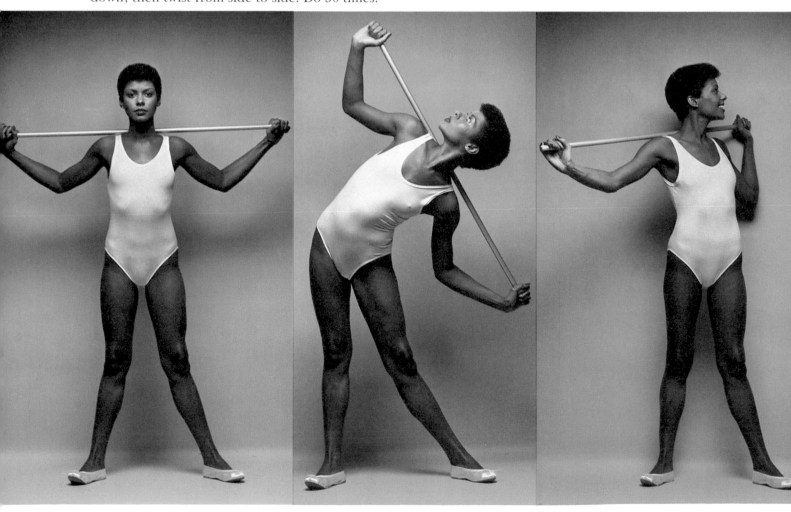

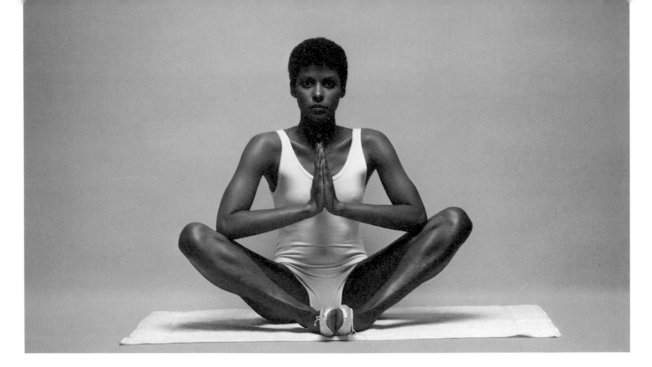

FOR THIGHS

Sit on the floor with your knees wide apart and the soles of your feet together. Put your palms together and press your elbows against your inner thighs. Push your legs together against the resistance of your arms. Hold for a slow count of 6; then relax for a slow count of 3. Reverse the force, with your elbows forcing your thighs outward. Hold for a slow count of 6; relax for a slow count of 3. Do 6 times.

Stand with your legs wide apart. Hold a broomstick upright, with both hands at the top end, and the bottom of the stick resting on the floor. Keeping your back straight and buttocks tucked in, knee-dip as far as you can to the left, then to the right. Do 12 times.

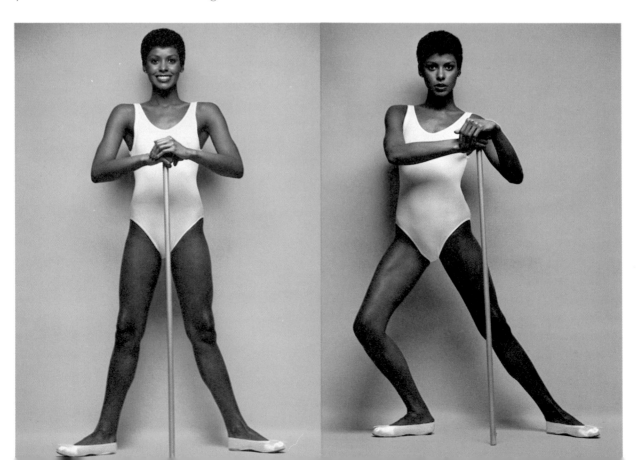

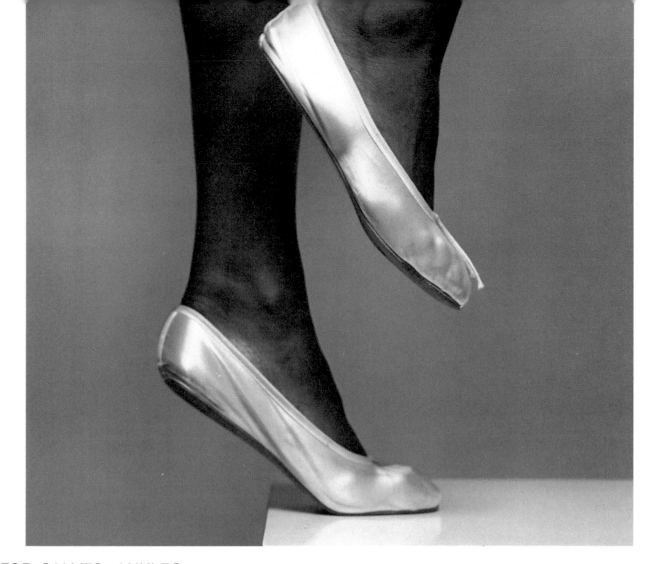

FOR CALVES, ANKLES

Keeping your back straight, tiptoe upstairs without letting your heels touch the stairs. At the top, relax. Holding on to the banister for balance, tiptoe downstairs backward.

Sit on an exercise mat or carpeted floor. Draw one knee toward your chest. Hold a broomstick near the ends with both hands and press the ball of the lifted foot against the stick. Then reverse the pressure by pressing the stick against the foot. Alternate legs and do 15 times for each leg.

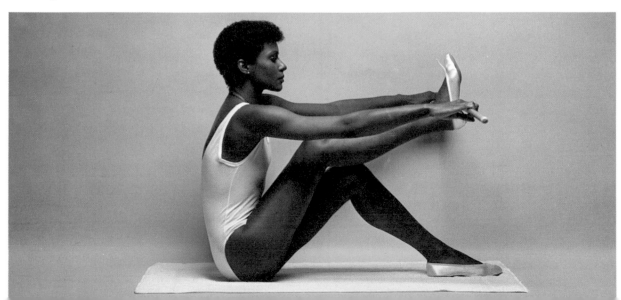

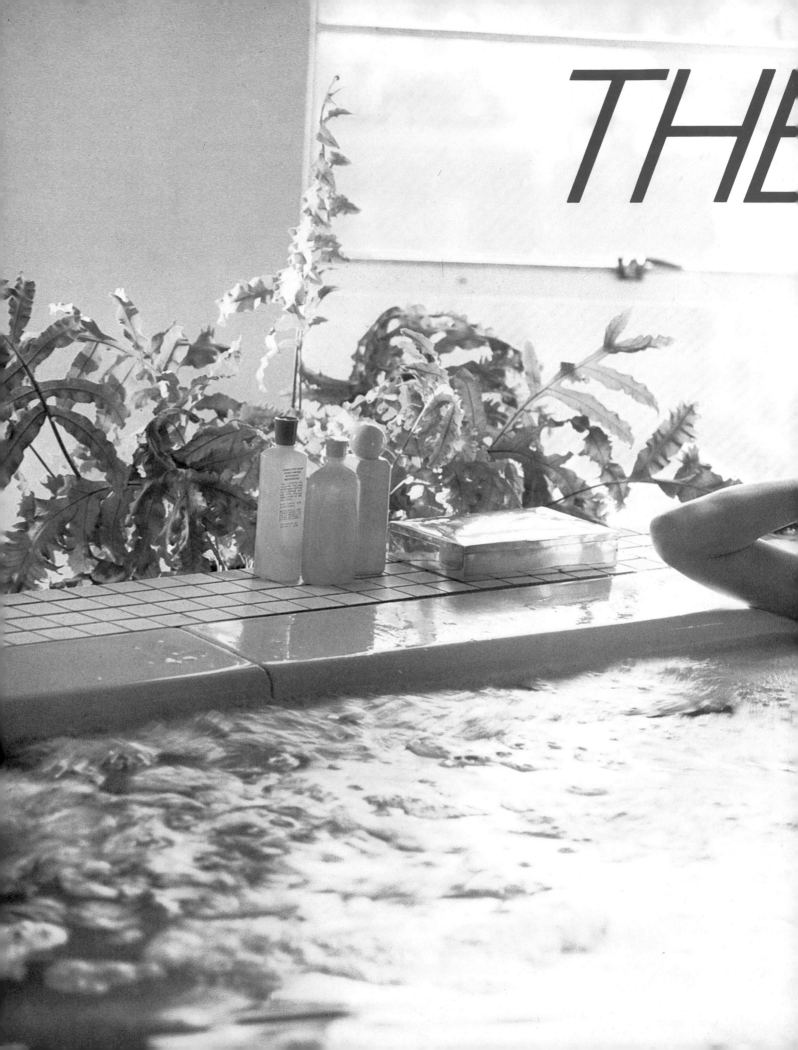

THE

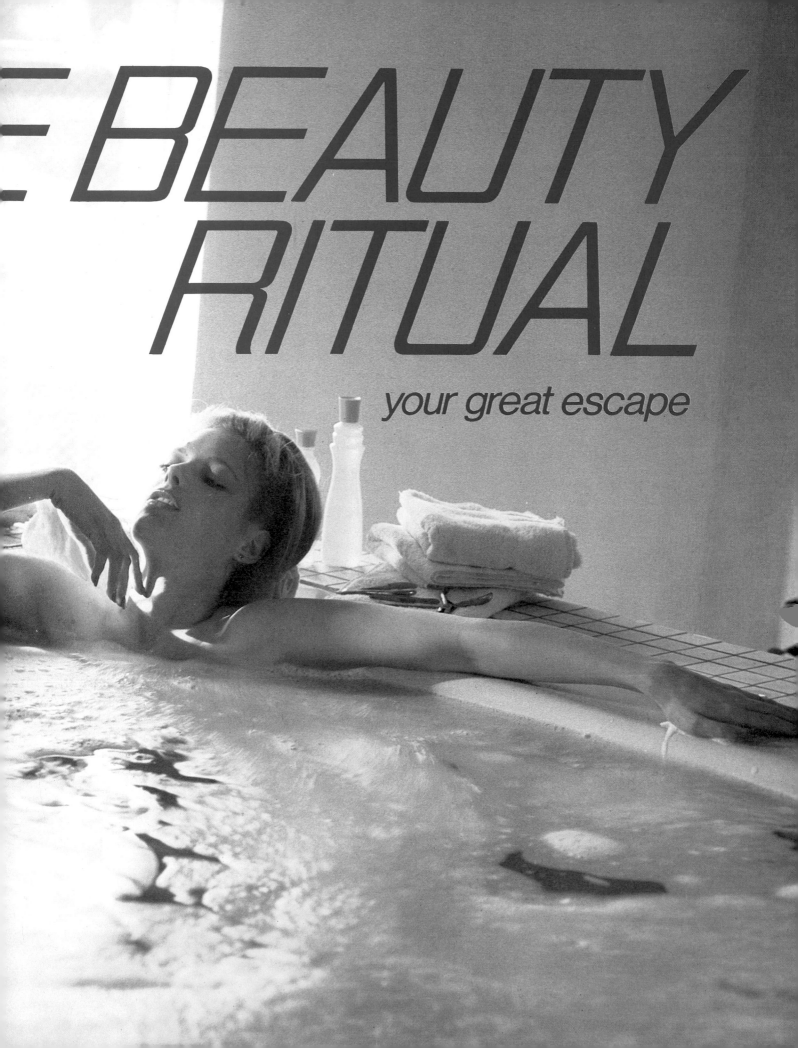

Make your bath your private spa

From the days of Cleopatra and Poppea, the bath has been the classic setting for beauty rituals. Throughout this book we've referred to "a warm, fragrant bath" as a beginning of each beauty checkup, and the reason is that it prepares you to think in terms of beauty. Even if you are a confirmed shower person, you owe yourself the weekly treat of at least one deliciously relaxing beauty bath.

Here's the suggested procedure for making the most of the bath and the beauty ritual as a part of the bath experience.

THE BEAUTY BATH

Set aside an hour or two during which you need have nothing on your mind but doing good things for yourself, small attentions that will make you look and feel prettier all week. Make the bath a joy for the senses—smell, sight, hearing, touch, and taste can all be enhanced by the bathing ritual.

1. Take a transistor radio into the bathroom and find a station that offers relaxing music without a lot of commercial interruptions or changes of program. Adjust to a low volume, set the radio in a safe, dry spot, and then begin your prebath beauty procedures.

2. Assemble everything you'll need for a manicure and pedicure (See pages 128 and 130). Remove old nail enamel and shape your nails with an emery board.

3. If you use a chemical depilatory or an electric razor to remove hair from legs and under arms, do this now before entering the bath. Rinse off all vestige of the cream before entering the bath.

4. Follow your usual plan for cleansing your face. You might want to apply a cleansing or moisturizing facial mask, or even your favorite moisturizer.

5. After you have shampooed your hair, use an instant conditioner, towel dry, and make a towel turban for your head. If you have used a conditioner that works over a longer time, cover your hair with a cap of clinging plastic kitchen wrap. To gain the advantage of heat's action on the conditioner, cover the plastic "cap" with a small towel soaked in hot water and then wrung out. Cover that with a terry-cloth turban.

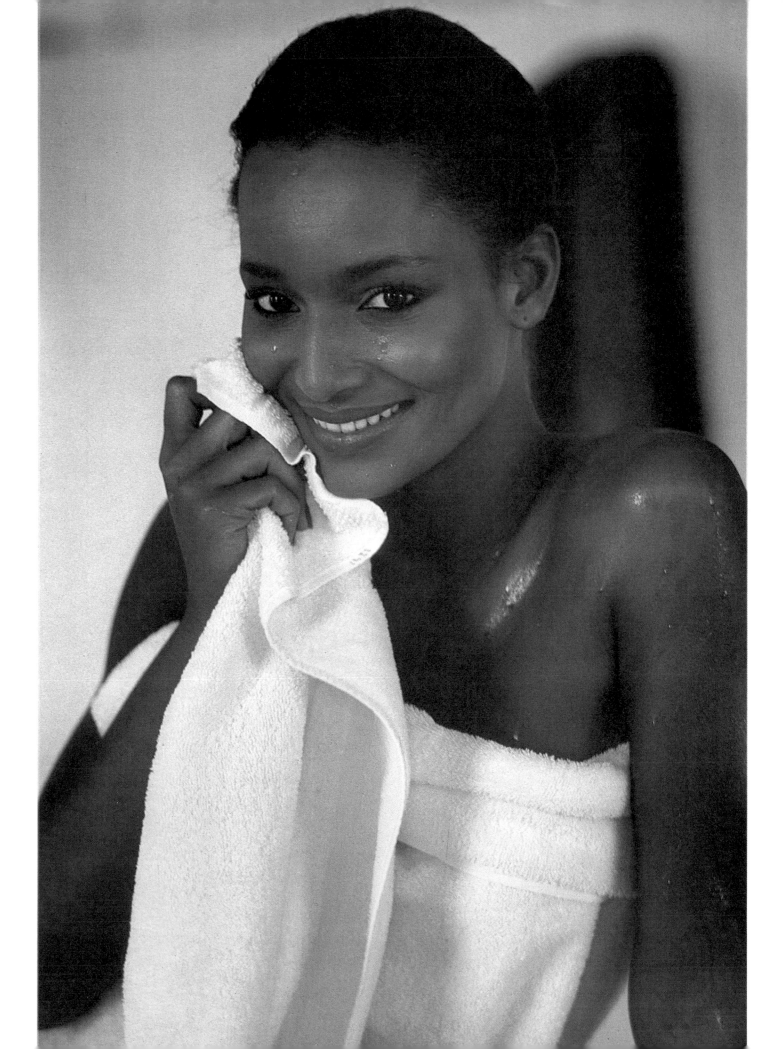

6. Draw the bath. The water should be warm, but not hot: body temperature is ideal. Test it as you would a baby's bottle—try a few drops of the bath water on the inside of your wrist, making sure it is neither hot nor cool to the touch. Add a dollop of skin-soothing bath gelée in your favorite fragrance; or pour luxurious bath oil into the water as the tub fills. Set out a couple of big, fluffy towels within your reach from the tub. Fold a third towel to form a cushion for your head while you soak, or use an air-filled plastic bath pillow. When the tub is a little more than half full, get into the bath and turn the warm water down to a trickle. This keeps the water temperature warm and constant while you soak, and the sound of running water will soothe your nerves.

7. Lie back and soak for about 10 minutes. Relax, unwind.

8. Rub a pumice stone on the rough areas of the body: the bottoms of your feet, and your elbows. Push back the cuticles of your nails. Scrub your fingernails and toenails with a nail brush.

9. Use a magnifying mirror and slant-edge tweezers to clean away any straggly growth on your eyebrows.

10. While you let the water out of the tub and run fresh warm water in, use a bath brush, a back brush, a loofah sponge, or other favorite means of scrubbing up a glowing skin all over your body.

11. If you have applied a facial mask, remove it now as directed; then splash your face with clear running water.

12. If you used a conditioning treatment on your hair, turn on the shower while the tub is draining and rinse out the conditioner.

13. Now is the time to shave your legs and underarms—if you use a safety razor. The warm bath has a softening effect on hair and makes shaving easier.

14. Step out of the tub and wrap yourself in a big, fresh towel to pat yourself dry. Smooth on a rich perfumed body moisturizer all over for fragrant, satiny skin. Follow with a light cloud of matching perfumed body talc, and put on a pretty, comfortable robe.

15. Now you begin with your pedicure (below).

16. Dry and style your hair.

17. Manicure: Directions for giving yourself a professional manicure can be found on page 130.

The 17-point plan above includes everything you might wish to include in your evening-long weekly Beauty Time. But don't feel you must do every single thing every single week. Instead, take from this master list only what's appropriate for your mood and the state of your looks this week. Next week you might want to spend more time on other areas. This might be the week for concentrated attention to your hair; next week you might want to lavish lots of care on a pedicure. Alter the program to suit your needs and your mood. But don't omit a part of your beauty ritual just because you forgot to allow enough time for a leisurely time of beauty. Stealing time away from this date with yourself is a real false economy.

THE PERFECT PEDICURE

1. Remove old nail enamel, as for a manicure. Clip toenails no shorter than the tips of toes, with edges squared, to discourage ingrown nails. File rough edges smooth with emery board. If nails are heavily ridged, smooth them with the smooth side of the emery board, or use a ridge filler (see step 3). Smooth cuticle remover around sides and base of the nails, and push cuticle back gently.

2. If you have not already accomplished this in the bath, soak your feet in warm, sudsy water. Scrub toenails and feet with a sudsy nail brush. To smooth away dead skin, calluses, and rough spots on heels and bottoms of the feet, use a wet pumice stone or a smoothing cream after drying your feet.

3. Dry your feet and gently push back cuticles. Fold tissue and weave it between toes, or use cotton balls, to separate toes. Apply base coat or a ridge filler to nails on the left foot; then do nails of the right foot while base coat dries. Apply a thin, even coat of nail enamel on nails of the left foot. Get as close to the cuticle as you can without actually covering

it. Now do the right foot. Alternating feet in this way gives enamel a longer drying time without actually taking up more of your time. Tidy up any smudges of enamel on skin with a cotton swab dipped in nail-enamel remover. Apply a second coat of enamel; then finish with top coat. When nails are dry, massage cream or lotion into your feet. Be lavish.

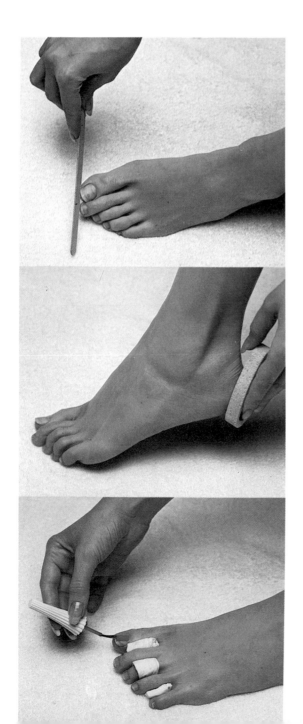

There's more to the walking-on-air feeling than just a pedicure. Below is a list of some of the things worth doing for your feet to help them do more for your outlook and your looks.

1. Slip off your shoes to give feet a breather during the day. Make it a real pleasure with refreshing footspray to cool you right through your stockings.

2. Walk barefoot when you can, but *only* on a springy surface—sand, thick grass, or wall-to-wall carpet. For hard surfaces, give your feet the protection of a resilient sole.

3. Wear heels of varying heights. Wearing the same heel height all the time can cause painful cramping of the calf muscle. And try not to wear the same shoes too many days in a row.

4. Shop for shoes in the early afternoon. Feet swell over the course of the day. Shoes bought late in the afternoon can be too loose next morning; bought in the morning, too tight that night.

5. Along with everything else about us, our feet change in size. There's even a difference in size between the right foot and the left. For a truly comfortable fit, have the salesperson measure both feet and choose the larger size. Stand while being measured, because the foot spreads when weight is applied, and you are buying shoes to stand and walk in, not merely to sit in.

6. Make sure panty hose are long enough. Stockings should fit with ½ inch to spare in the toes.

7. Pull out the toe of your stocking before slipping on shoes.

8. Ask around for the name of a good podiatrist, and keep the number handy. Call at the first hint of foot trouble. A red spot on the toe is such a hint. A corn is starting to form. Act now.

9. Feet swell when you sit for a long time, especially on a plane. Get out of your seat and walk if you can. If you can't, rotate your ankles, flex your legs, curl your toes and stretch them.

10. Prop up your feet whenever you can. Even a few minutes with feet elevated helps.

11. Strengthen arches by standing pigeon-toed and rising on toes. Do this four or five times in succession whenever it occurs to you.

12. Alternate very warm and icy cold foot baths or use a refreshing foot spray if you really want to rev up tired feet and relieve soreness.

13. Massage your feet whenever there's an opportunity. Knead them, working up from toes to the calves.

14. Feet also benefit from moisturizing. Never forget to cream your feet with body lotion after a shower or bath. Dust them with talcum before putting on stockings.

INVEST A LITTLE
TIME IN YOUR HANDS

Her manicure—or lack of one—spoiled things for Scarlett O'Hara. The splendid effect of her new curtain dress was ruined when Rhett saw her callused hands. In real life too, people notice hands quickly. Hands that are beautifully cared for say you care for yourself and others. And they make quite a statement about your fashion sense when nails are shapely and colorful.

A weekly manicure is a must for pretty hands. Borrow the professional manicure techniques used in expensive salons, and you will find the procedure is simple and speedy.

SALON MANICURE AT HOME

For speed and convenience, assemble everything you will use before you begin. And give yourself a good, focused work light. You'll need:

bowl of warm, sudsy water	cotton pads
	orange stick
emery board	nail brush
nail enamel remover	ridge filler
cuticle clipper	base coat
cuticle conditioner	top coat
nail strengthener	nail enamel
cuticle remover	nail enamel dryer
	hand towel

1. Soak cotton pad with nail enamel remover. Press down on nail, using a rocking motion of your thumb on cotton pad to take up all the old enamel; then whisk it off quickly. This gives a cleaner removal than rubbing the nail; also, less remover is apt to get into the cuticle. If necessary, repeat to remove every trace of old nail enamel.

2. File dry nails with an emery board. File toward center of nail in one direction only; don't saw. Shape nails into slightly blunted ovals to discourage splits.

3. Soak fingertips for a minute or two in warm, sudsy water to resoften cuticle and wash away traces of remover. Rinse and dry hands.

4. Smooth cuticle remover into sides and base of each nail. Let it work for a minute or so. Push back cuticles gently.

5. Dip fingers into warm, sudsy water and brush. If you have a hangnail, use the cuticle clipper to remove the torn skin. Don't clip into the cuticle itself—that encourages more hangnails!

6. Massage cuticle conditioner around the base and sides of each nail. This keeps cuticle strong and pliable to protect nails, and discourages splitting and hangnails. Rinse off excess.

7. Clean, dry nails are now ready for nail strengthener to firm and seal nails against splits, chips, and breaks. Hold brush so it spreads out flat against the nail. A thin, even coat adheres best.

8. Follow with a base coat applied the same way. A base coat helps nail enamel flow on smoother, cling longer.

9. Apply nail enamel in two thin coats, letting enamel dry between coats. Spread each coat sparingly—one dip of the brush will be enough for one nail. Put down each coat in three smooth strokes from base to tip of nail. Stroke down the center first, then each side.

10. Shield your finished manicure with a thin, even coat of glossy top coat. It adds beautiful gleaming protection so nails look better all week long. Between manicures, you may want to apply fresh top coat every few days. It's a good idea for lasting power and gloss.

11. Apply a nail-enamel dryer to help prevent smearing while enamel dries.

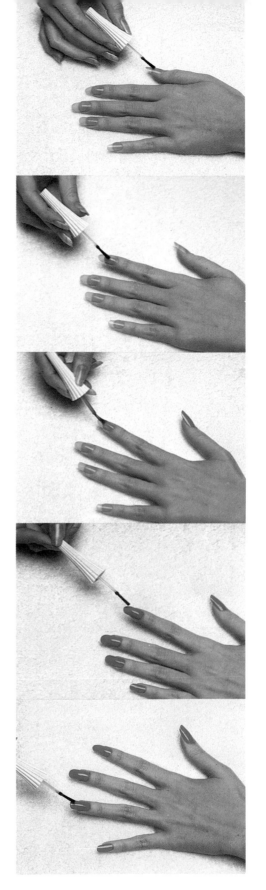
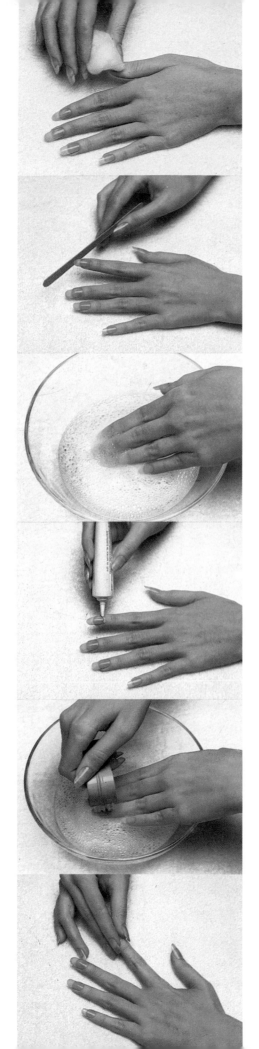

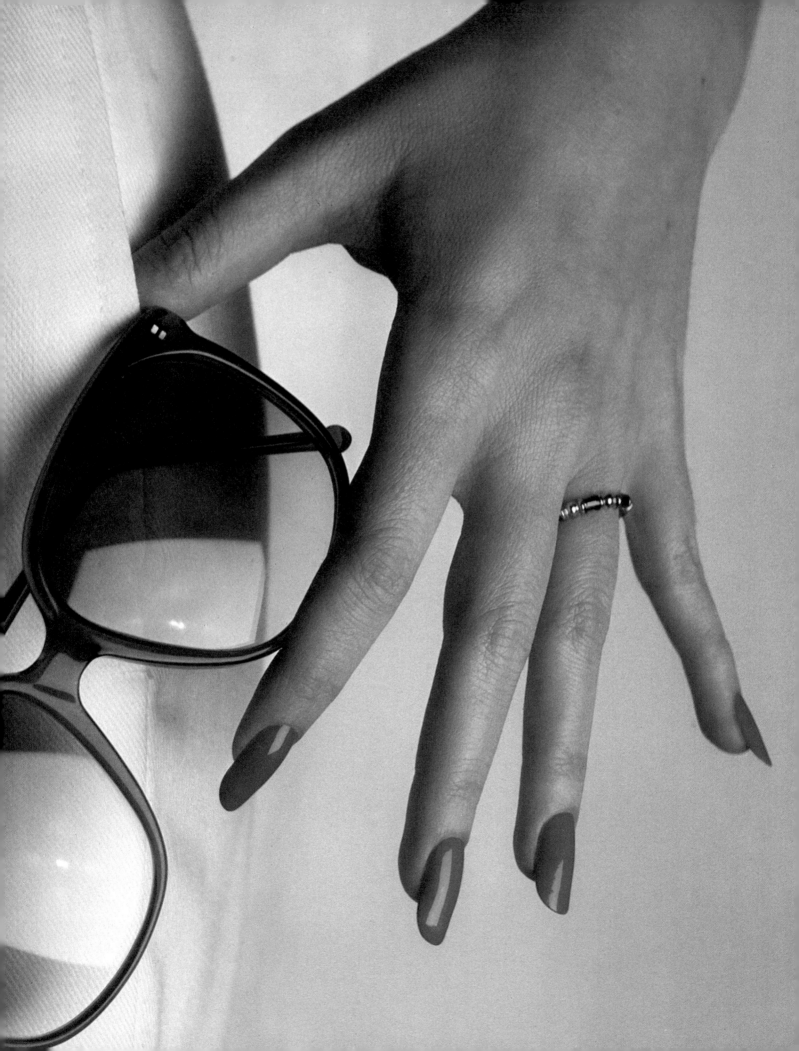

Beautiful nails

HOW TO GROW THEM AND
HOW TO KEEP THEM

A list of tips and nail facts to have on hand:
- Nails grow constantly. But the nail you see has already done its growing and is just being pushed along by the new, living nail that is formed down in the nail bed below the skin. The part you see is only about half the nail. You can see only the very tip of the other half—the matrix—and that tip is called the "moon." Proteins and trace minerals are transformed in the matrix into a proteinlike substance called keratin. Your cuticles serve as a kind of weather seal to protect the nail bed from infection.
- Three to six months are needed for a whole new nail to form. Average growth is about an eighth of an inch per month. But nails grow slightly faster in hot weather, on the middle fingers, and on the right hand for right-handed people. Circulation helps, too. Your nails grow a little faster if you play the piano, or type, or massage your fingers up from knuckles to tips.
- The way your nails grow is a question of heredity, exercise, nutrition, and overall health. But you can take on-the-spot measures to help them. *Brittle* nails benefit from massaging with cuticle conditioner. *Soft* nails improve if kept protected by rubber gloves whenever hands come in contact with hot water and detergent. *Peeling* nails could be a result of fungus. See your doctor.
- Nail enamel is easier to work with, goes farther, and lasts longer if you: shake the closed bottle well before opening (air bubbles won't form) stroke the brush against inside rim of the bottle before applying to nails; wipe the inside of the bottle cap with a cotton pad dampened in nail-enamel remover before replacing the cap (the top will never stick).
- Exposing the half moons and covering the rest of the nail with enamel is a look that keeps coming back into fashion. It does tend to make nails look shorter, but you may enjoy the fanciful effect. Here's how: stroke on polish like an inverted T. Center-stroke from middle of the nail to tip; next, the cross stroke from one side of nail to the other to form the moon. Finally, fill in the sides.
- Nails need at least two coats of enamel, but many manicurists keep right on going with as many as six thin coats! They say it enriches the deep-down gleam as well as the protection.
- Keep nails out of water as much as possible for the first day after manicuring. Definitely avoid hot water at all times. It is bad for your skin as well as your nails. If you wash dishes by hand, wear rubber gloves and use a dishwashing brush to keep hands above the water line as much as possible. Let dishes soak in very hot sudsy water; then come back to finish them off when water has cooled. Go about another task during their soak time. This is easier on hands and nails, takes no longer, and even eases removal of soil from the dishes.
- Apply a coat of top coat or strengthener every other day to keep your manicure in great condition. If you do this, you may be able to go as long as two weeks between manicures.
- You get an even better manicure if you do it in short sessions rather than one take. At night, do your manicure through the first coat of nail enamel. Next morning, apply the second coat of enamel. Later in the day, apply top coat. Result: only seconds here and there of your time, but lots of drying time for nail enamel. And nail enamel that is dried thoroughly between coats never bubbles and resists chips.
- Don't use nails as rakes or shovels. If you must poke around in your handbag or a drawer, use the eraser end of a pencil, not your index finger. Form the habit of using the flat side of your palm instead of your

fingertips for such tasks as sweeping up coins from a tabletop. Use the eraser end of a pencil to dial or press the buttons on a telephone. Use your knuckle, not your nail, to ring the doorbell or summon the elevator. Pry open a jewelry clasp with a metal nail file, not your nail.

■ Buffing gently is good for nails. If you choose not to wear nail enamel, buffing is a must for softly gleaming nails. A dozen strokes should be plenty.

■ Here's a trick with top coat that will disguise a small nick in nail enamel. Apply top coat on the damaged nail. Let it set for a few seconds; then slowly stroke over the chipped spot. You will loosen a little enamel color to blend by doing this, and the chip will be disguised.

■ Rubber gloves should be comfortably loose and should be cotton-lined. A loose fit permits air circulation, so hands stay cooler and drier, and an absorbent lining prevents hands from being bathed in perspiration. Wear gloves whenever doing wet or dirty chores, but remove them as soon as you're done so hands can stay cool and dry.

■ Keep cuticle conditioner in your purse and use it to keep busy when you find yourself in a sitting-and-waiting situation. Travel time to and from work is a good time to massage a little conditioner around the sides and the base of the nail. It doesn't damage your manicure or affect your nail enamel in any way, but it will help keep your cuticles soft and prevent splitting and hangnails.

■ Keep a tube or bottle of hand cream in every place where you are likely to get your hands wet—bathroom, kitchen, laundry room, wherever. Use cream on your hands before putting them in water. After drying them, cream again, and always remember to push cuticle back gently when you dry.

■ If you pinch a nail in a drawer or a door, raise your hand immediately to prevent a rush of blood to the area, and apply a cold compress as quickly as possible.

■ A broken nail can be mended, and protected from further splitting. You can buy kits with nail-mending papers and liquid; follow instructions carefully.

■ Clear enamel will help protect and beautify nails, but don't pass up the fun of making a fashion statement with color. A pretty color calls attention to well-shaped nails and flatters the skin. It's also an accessory and color accent for your costume. Deep rich colors complement very dark skin tones. Unless they contrast with skin tone, deep colors also make the nail look smaller. Brighter colors accentuate longer nails. Nail color that is closely related to skin color helps make hands look long and slender and even helps disguise short nails. It is also lots of fun to coordinate nail and lip color.

REMOVING BODY HAIR

Fuzzy skin is lovely. On a peach. A certain fuzziness or hairiness is a universal human characteristic. But in this country, at least, we think a well-groomed woman's legs and underarms should be sleek. Quite a lot of time and thought have gone into the best way to bare skin. There are many methods: bleaching to camouflage; tweezing, waxing, and electrolysis to uproot the hair; depilation to dissolve the hair with chemicals; and shaving to cut off hair growth at the skin line.

Shaving and depilation are far and away the most common and practical methods for hair removal. Here's a quick take on the range of options open to you in the battle against hair on the body and face. (Tweezing is for eyebrows only. Tips on the best way are in the Makeup chapter.)

Bleaching: not really a hair-removal method, but one to make hair much less visible. Used on the face, forearms, and body. A chemical bleach strips color from the hair. Especially good for women with dark hair on their upper lips or sideburns. It takes time and careful work. A skin-patch test the day before bleaching is a must, and dark hair may require two bleach sessions one day apart. Facial hair will then require weekly touch-ups. Use a good commercial bleaching preparation and follow directions.

Depilation: uses a chemical depilatory to dissolve hair above and below skin surface. Used on arms, underarms, legs, body, and—sometimes—the face. Depilatory use is painless. However, chemicals that are strong enough to dissolve hair are strong enough to harm some types of skin. A first-time skin-patch test the day before using is vital. If your skin is not irritated, you can proceed with depilation. But depilatories can be messy and slippery enough to constitute a safety hazard when used in the tub. Sit on the edge of the tub with your feet in the tub, and keep lukewarm water running so you can rinse often to keep the job as neat as possible. Follow package instructions carefully.

Electrolysis: uses electric current to render the hair follicle sterile. Current is transmitted through a platinum or steel stylus inserted in a pore. Used on face, breasts, and abdominal hair. It hurts (some women find the pain intolerable; others scarcely notice it). It takes time, as only a certain number of hairs can be sterilized in each session, and some very strong follicles may require more than one electric shock. It must be done professionally. This method of hair removal is expensive, so be well warned. Should you wish to investigate electrolysis, check with your family doctor or dermatologist as well as the Better Business Bureau.

Shaving: is quick and inexpensive. It does not harm hair, nor does it, as some people still believe, stimulate hair growth. This myth grew up because regrowth of blunt-cut hair seems more bristly than the naturally tapering growth of virgin hair. Used for legs and underarms only. Never shave forearms or hair on the face. The smoothest, neatest job—with no nicks or drying of the skin—results if you always use a fresh blade; never use anything but a special shaving cream or foam shave; never use a razor without using water and shave foam to soften hair, make it elastic and easy to remove; rinse the razor after every stroke—hair and shaving cream clog the razor and lead to skipped patches and nicks.

Electric razors work best if you apply pre-shave conditioner to the skin; use short, separate pressing strokes of the electric razor instead of long, sweeping ones.

Many women feel that switching back and forth each week from electric to manual razors is easier on the skin.

Either way, rinse well after shaving and apply lots of soothing, moisturizing lotion.

How often you shave depends entirely on the rate of hair growth. You might need to shave every two weeks, or twice a day. No matter how often you shave, shaving will not cause more hair to grow. Hair can grow only where there is a hair follicle, and you have all the hair follicles you ever will have at birth. You can't grow more hair follicles by shaving.

Waxing: has some good arguments for and against. Pros include no stubble of regrowth, no chemical injury to the skin or hair follicle. Cons are that it's expensive, it's time-consuming, and it hurts—a little or a lot, depending on the sensitivity of the part of the body and your own threshold of pain. It also can cause ingrown hairs. Waxing works best if you allow a longer time between sessions than you would with other methods, so that there is enough hair to give the wax a grip. Beeswax is heated, spread in the direction of hair growth, covered with muslin strips; then, after a few minutes, pulled off, as you would strip off a bandage. The hair comes out along with the wax. A simple process, but one best left to a professional. If you try to wax at home, follow directions carefully.

Now that you are refreshed from your bath —your skin clean, smooth, and glowing—you are ready for the final step that will enhance and intensify your new beauty personality.

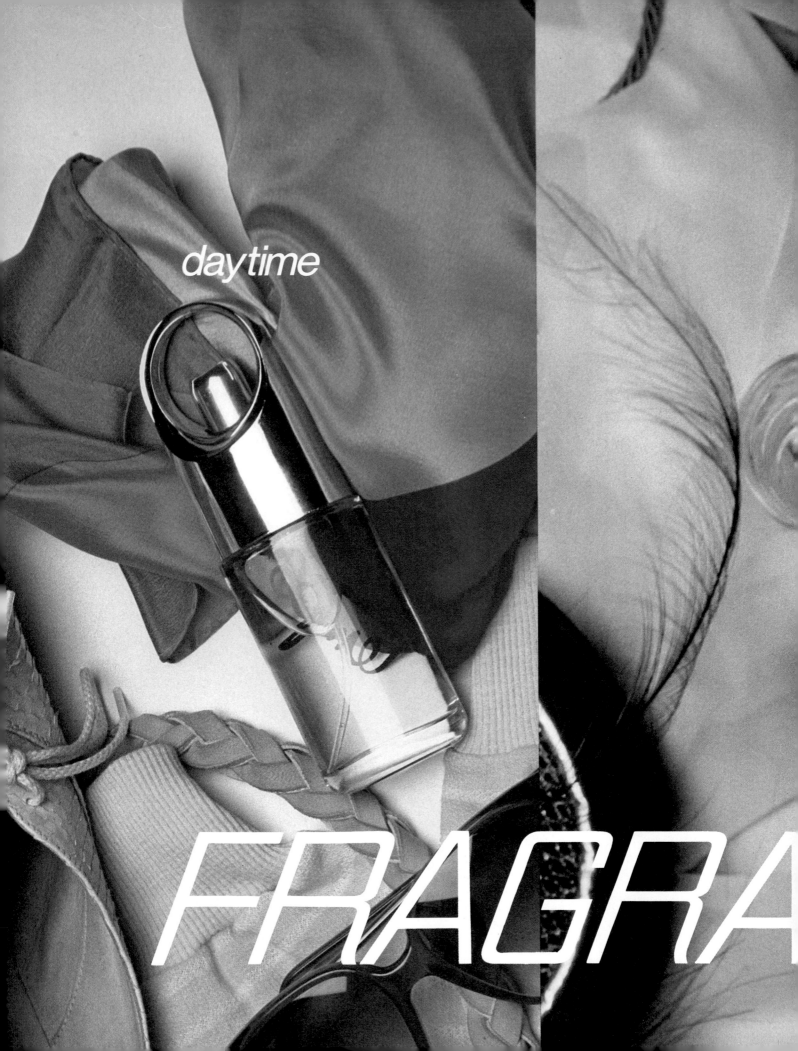

daytime

FRAGRA

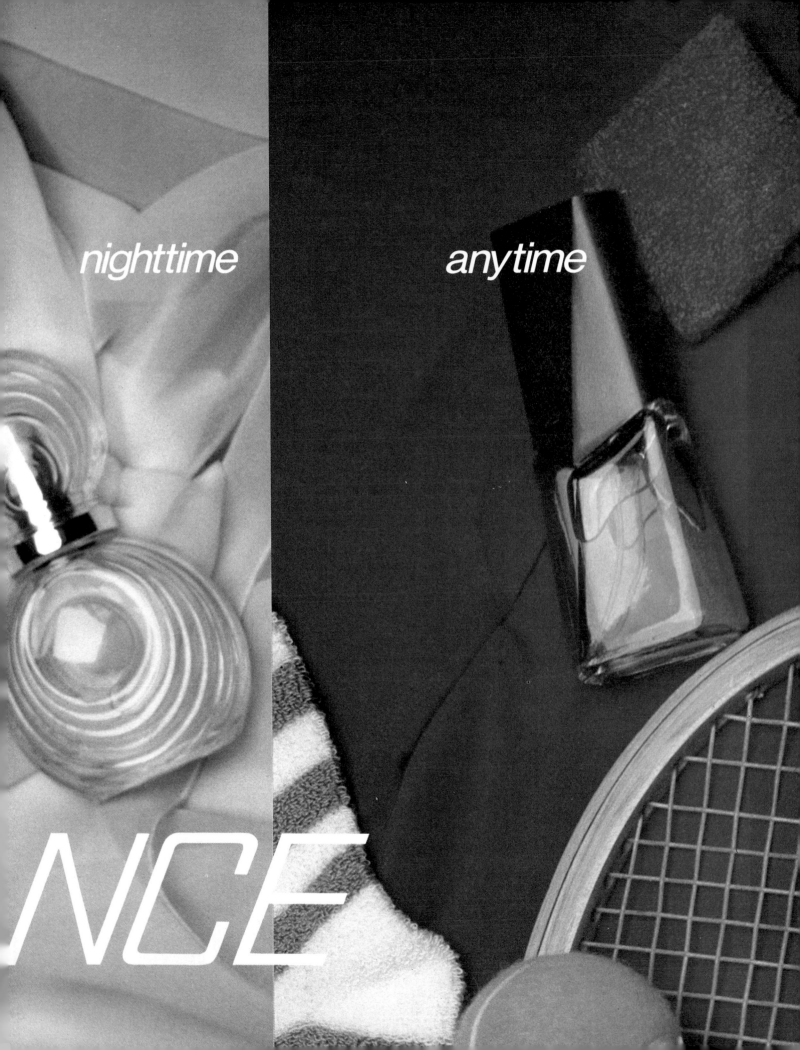

nighttime

anytime

NCE

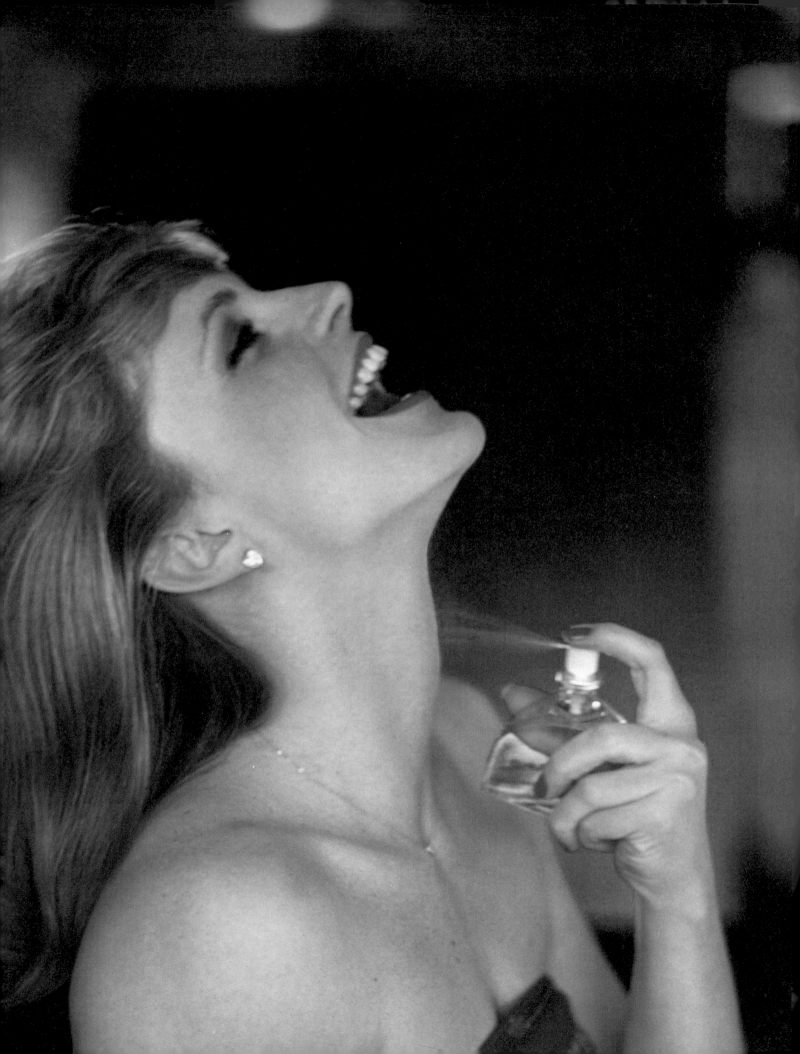

Fragrance

Now you're feeling beautiful.

If you have followed the suggestions in this book so far, you will notice a remarkable change in your appearance. Your hair will be softer and shinier; your complexion will look clearer and more radiant; your eyes will be brighter and more sparkling—even your toenails will be more shapely.

And now that you've come this far, we will share with you one of the most important and most subtle beauty secrets of them all. We will talk about how to create your own aura and mystique, a memorable impression that softly lingers after you have left the room. The secret is *fragrance*.

Fragrance in all its delightful variety has always been an important echo of femininity, but today fragrance has become an absolutely essential part of the modern woman's fashion planning. From this day on, your fragrance must be thought of as an indispensable addition to your beauty personality.

At one time perfume was reserved for Special Occasions Only, like wearing a floor-length evening dress, and a woman was given one special "signature fragrance" that she used to commemorate important evenings. But the modern woman sees her whole life as a series of special occasions and knows that variety is the spice of life. Now she buys and wears fragrance every day and every night creates a wardrobe of scents as versatile as the clothing she wears.

Today we spray or dab on colognes and perfumes to make us feel fresher and prettier all day, every day. Different fragrances help reflect our varied moods, the different facets of our personalities. We can collect an entire wardrobe of perfumes and colognes to complement our wardrobe of clothing; we can don the proper scent no matter what the season, sport, or social event.

Because of the enormous range of ingredients that are available to the perfumer, fragrances can match your changing mood even if you are, like Cleopatra, a woman of "infinite variety." Part scientist but mostly artist, the perfumer combines, blends, mixes and merges thousands of ingredients until he finds the scent that evokes the image and mood for which he is searching.

Although innumerable notes make up the spectrum, the perfumer draws upon six basic groups of ingredients.

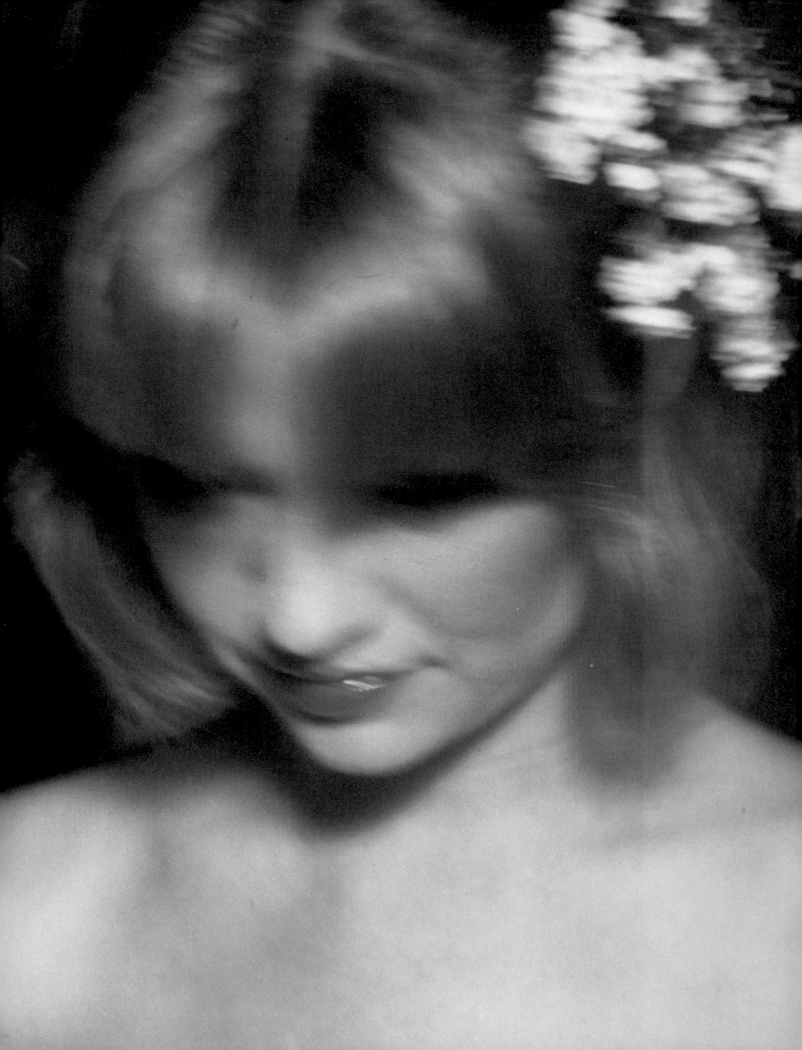

The Six Great Families of Fragrance

Single Florals

—capture the essence of a single blossom.

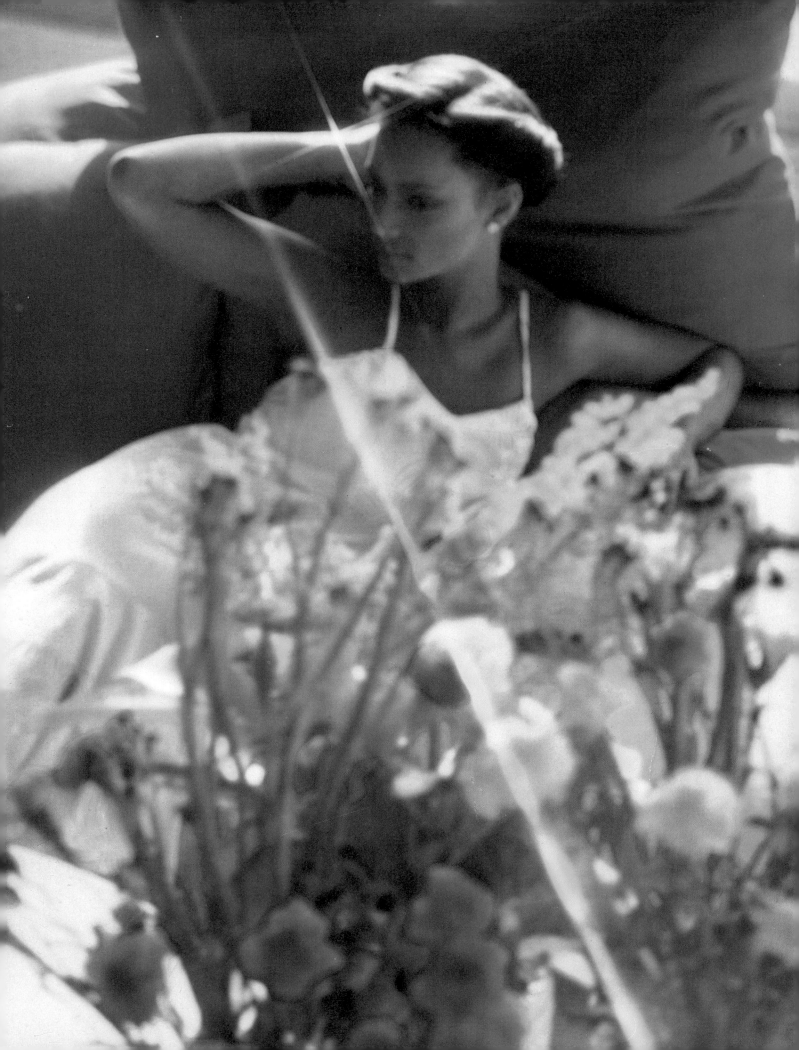

The Six Great Families of Fragrance

Floral Bouquets

—blend a bouquet of different flower notes
into an intricate and subtle harmony. It may
not be easy to identify the specific flowers
combined, but the fragrance is definitely
"flowery" in character.

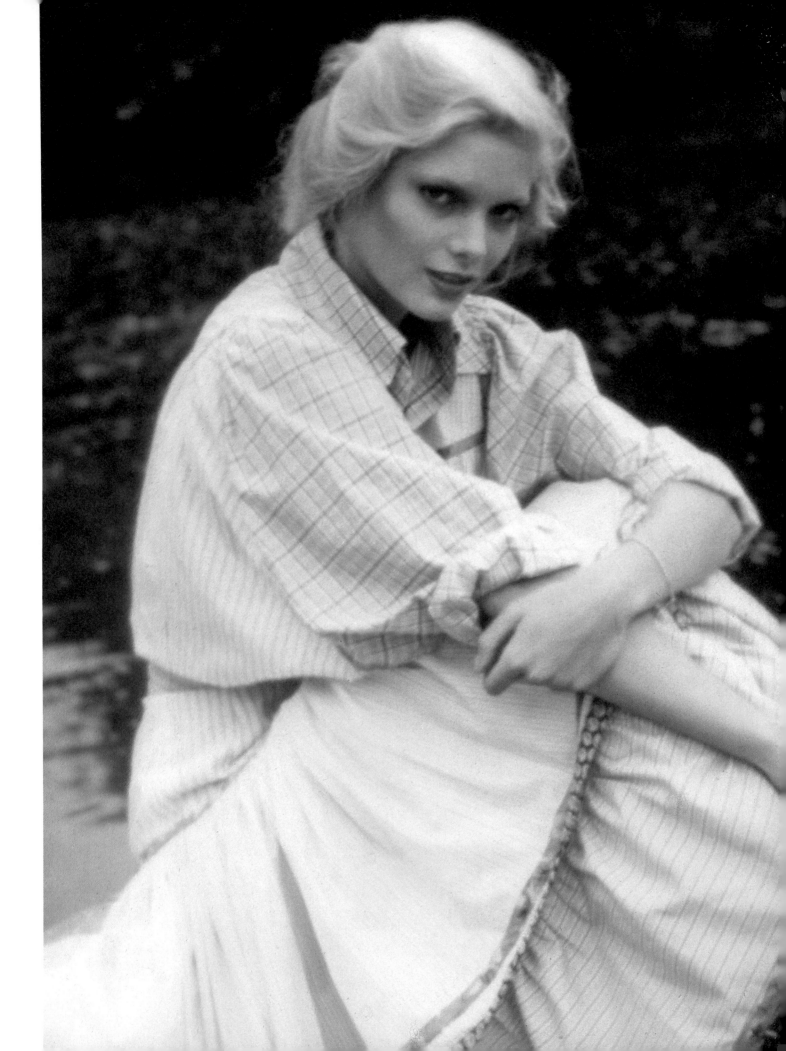

The Six Great Families of Fragrance

Leafy, Woodsy, Mossy Blends

—combine aromatic woods, such as cedar, with the aromas of flower stems, leaves, ferns, oakmoss and other herbal scents for a clean, refreshing fragrance with a "foresty" appeal.

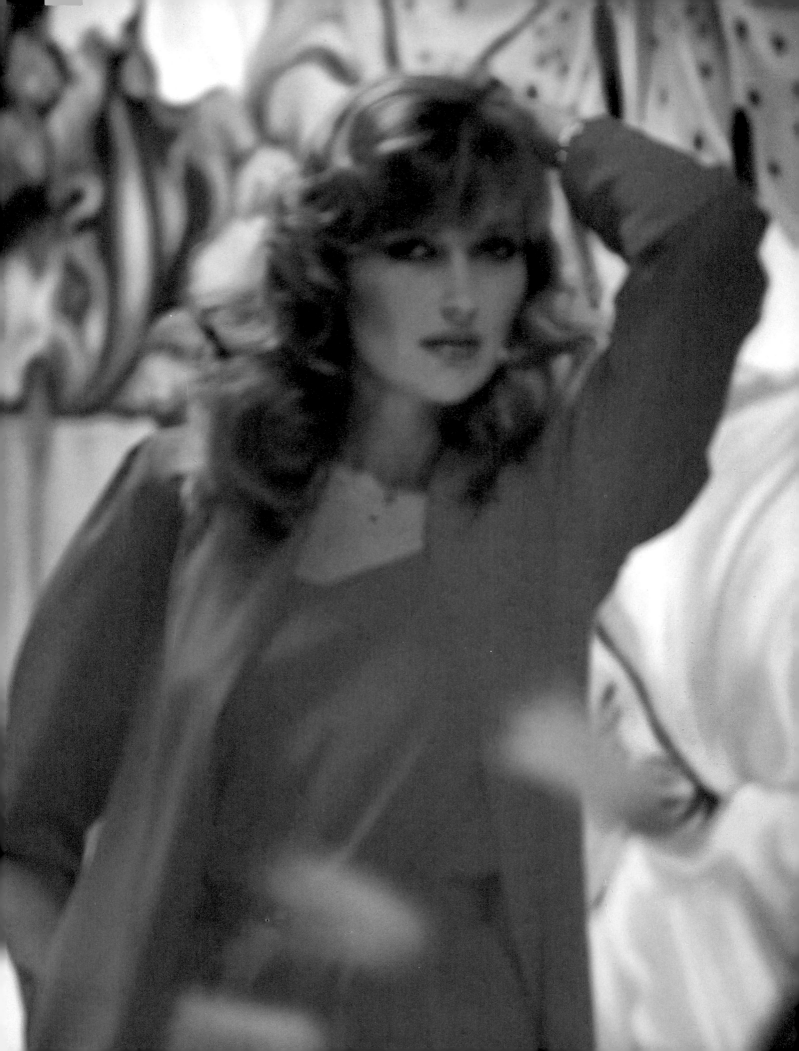

Spicy, Fruity Blends

—meld the clean, fresh quality of citrus fruits and pungent spices such as clove, cinnamon or ginger with, perhaps, spicy flower aromas such as carnation, and hints of mellow, peachlike warmth. These are apt to be sparkling, outdoorsy fragrances, light and fresh, but they may shade down into rich, full-bodied fragrances.

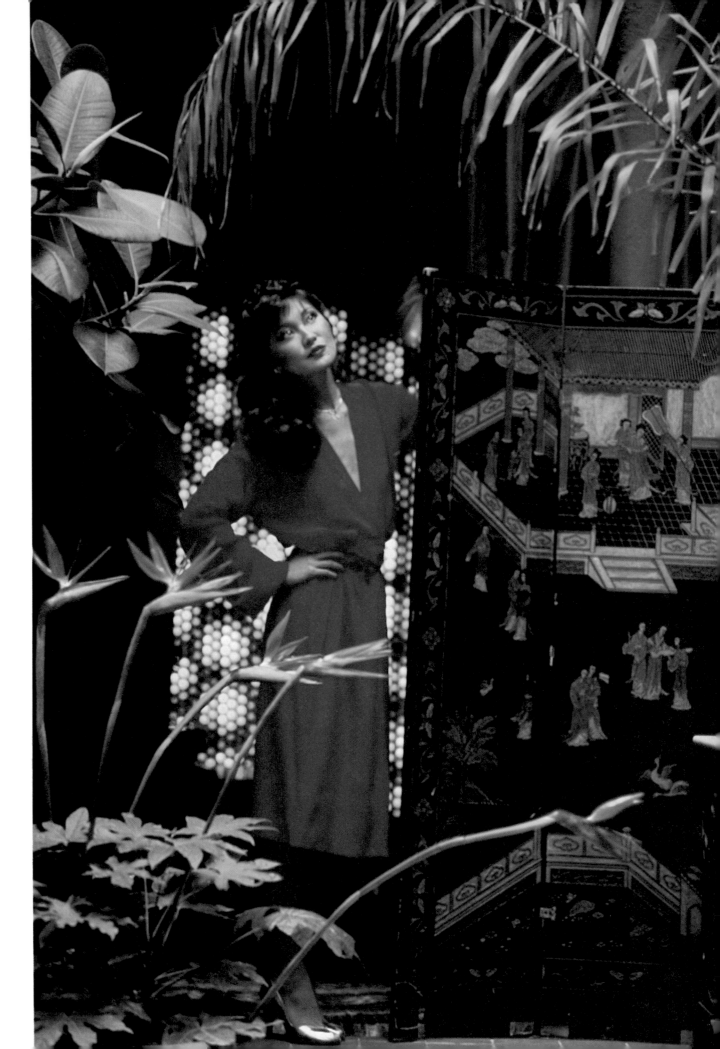

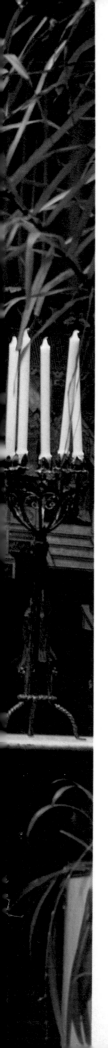

The Six Great Families of Fragrance

Oriental Blends

—evoke the mystery and richness of the Orient
through sophisticated combinations of musk
and amber along with many exotic blossoms.
These blends are apt to be haunting, intense,
and sweet or smoky.

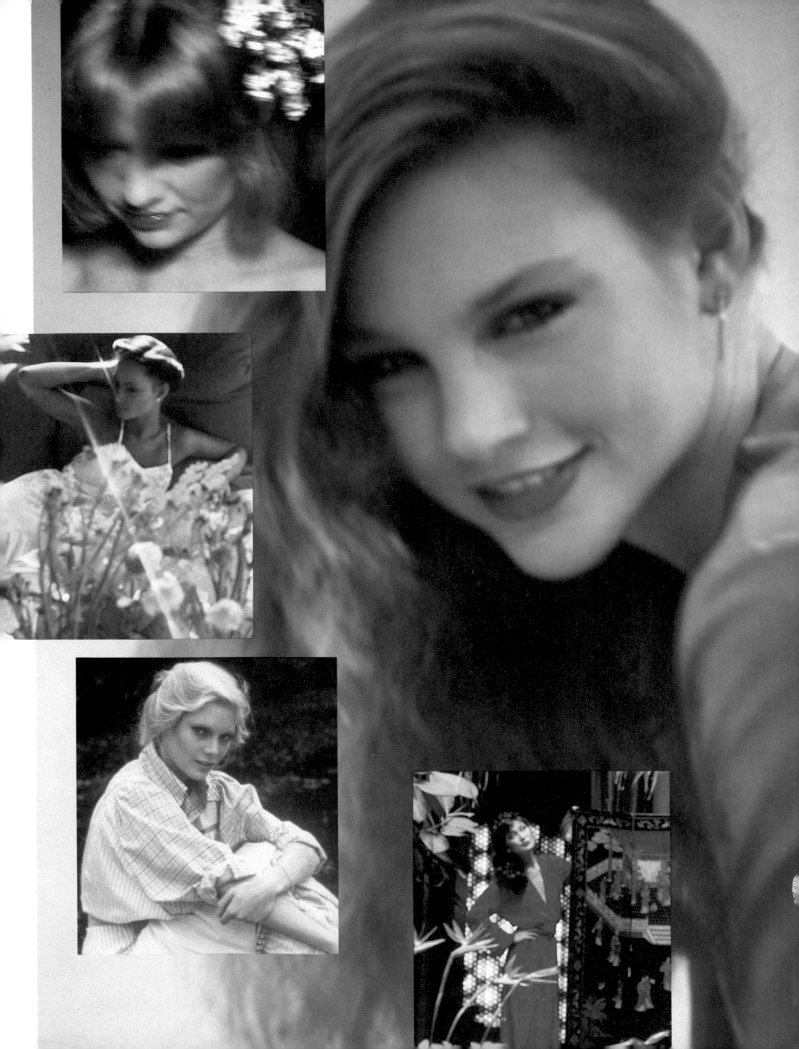

Modern Blends

—may contain notes from any or all other fragrance categories, yet they do not duplicate anything in nature. Rather, these are sparkling new creations of the perfumer. They have a full-bodied total impact that is characterized by a brilliant sparkle.

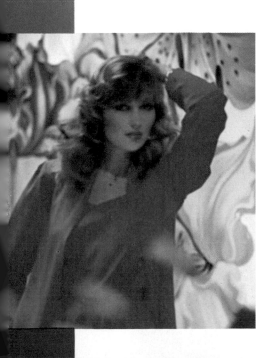

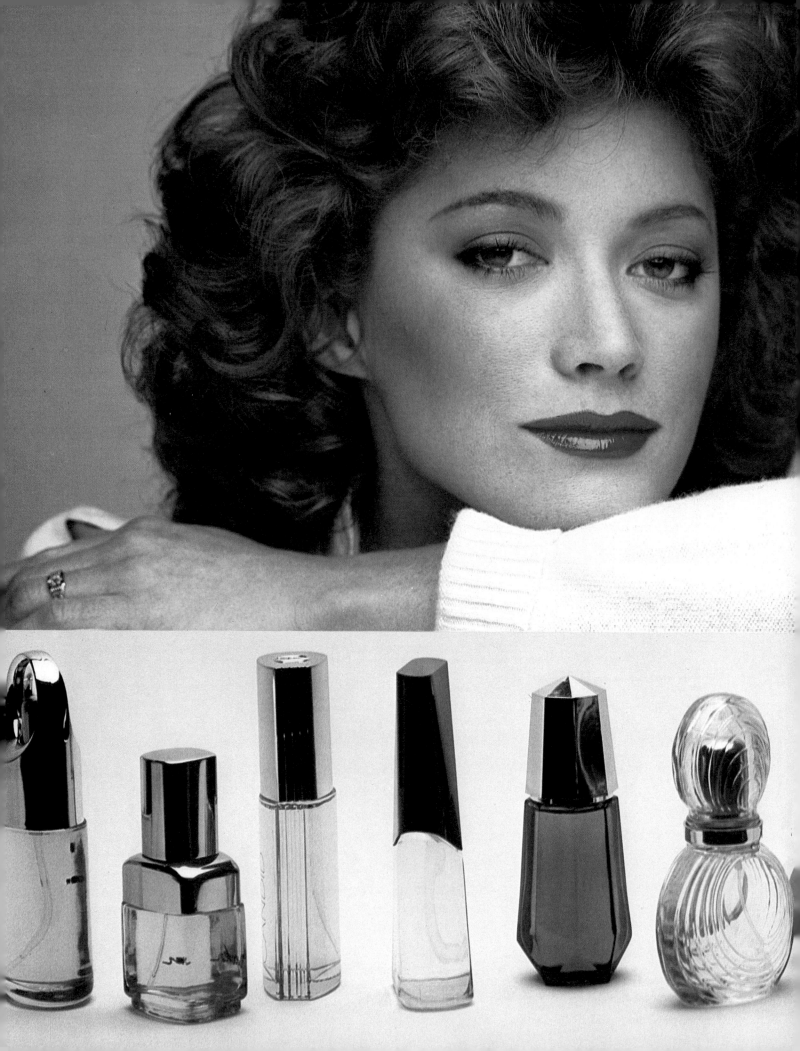

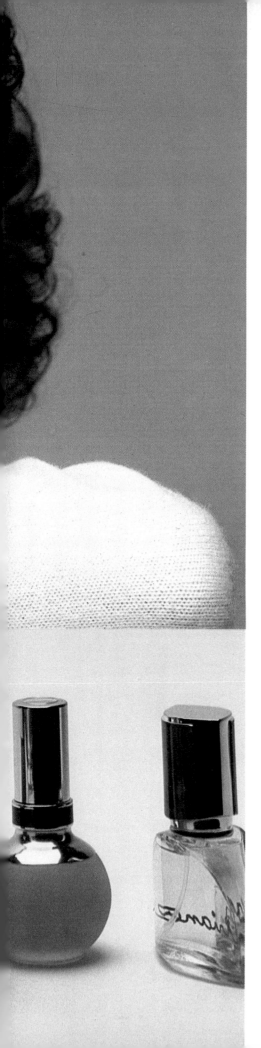

Most women are delighted when they see many different fragrances in beautifully shaped containers, with elegant ribbons, pastel-colored wrappings, and exotic names that evoke faraway places or passionate romance. But how do you choose the right scent for you?

Although each fragrance, with its exquisite packaging and exotic name, cries out, "Buy Me!" the way it is advertised can nonetheless be a real clue to the scent you are searching for. Scents do suggest moods—a "green" fragrance evokes the freshness of the country; a musk, a sense of intimacy and romance; lemon, a hint of summer breezes—and manufacturers are quick to name their scents and write their ads in accordance with these psychological associations. An ad that shows a tennis match, for example, tells you that the perfume featured has a light, informal quality, whereas the ad picturing a couple holding hands in the moonlight suggests an intense, intimate aroma.

But no matter what the ad, or your friends, say, the only sure way to find a fragrance is to experiment. Get set for an adventure—and don't be afraid to experiment.

When testing a scent, keep in mind that you cannot really tell how a fragrance smells by sniffing it out of the bottle. Even when it is on your skin, a scent will actually change within the first ten minutes of application.

The immediate perception or first impression of a scent is called the "top note." Soon the full fragrance will begin to unfold. This stage is referred to as the "middle note," or "heart." The full character, or long-term impression, of a scent is not discernible until several minutes after application, when it has had time to blend with the natural oils of the skin. The fragrance is altered at this stage by your individual chemistry, which provides the missing note—and makes that fragrance distinctly your own. Perfumers call this stage "dry-down." Other people slowly become aware of your fragrance as the warmth of your skin helps the scent radiate outward. This process is called diffusion.

THE FORMS OF FRAGRANCE

LIQUIDS: The most traditional form of fragrance is liquid. Cologne is perfume oil in an alcohol base. It comes in varying strengths depending upon the concentration of perfume oils. The ultra-colognes have the greatest strength and are the most long-lasting.

Perfume is composed of the highest concentration of perfume oils. It is generally the most expensive and richest form of a fragrance.

PUMP SPRAYS: These are liquid fragrances that are drawn up through a tube and forced out through a small opening in the top. The mist created by the spray covers a wider area of the skin than ordinary liquid fragrances and results in greater diffusion.

CREAMS: Creams, lotions and glacé fragrances take longer to diffuse than liquid forms, because the warmth of the skin is necessary to release the fragrance.

OILS: Perfume oils are highly concentrated fragrance in an oil base. They are exceedingly long-lasting and very intense in aroma.

6 BEAUTIFUL WAYS TO CREATE A FRAGRANCE WARDROBE

1. Use your sense of timing. Tests show that the sense of smell grows more acute as the day goes on. Your power is at its peak in the late afternoon. That's the golden hour for testing.

2. Pick your spot. The inside of the wrist, where the pulse beats close to the surface, and the back of the wrist are ideal proving grounds for a drop or light spray of fragrance.

3. Narrow the field. Try one perfume on the right wrist, one on the left. Don't try to juggle more than two fragrances at a time. Our noses become confused, scientists say, by too many scents at a time: our minds mix them all together. When there are too many temptations around to content yourself with sampling only two, try this: Take a quick sniff of the perfumed soap that matches a fragrance. You won't get the true sense of how the fragrance will work on you, but you will be able to decide whether or not you like the basic idea without paralyzing your sense of smell. But limit even this preliminary sampling to no more than four at a session.

4. Don't rush it. Give perfume and your skin a chance to get acquainted and interact. Remember it takes several minutes before fragrance develops fully on your skin.

5. Explore your individuality. Each skin's chemistry is unique, so perfume never smells exactly the same on any two women. Explore and exploit this lovely way of being yourself. Always sample a fragrance by the way it smells on *you* before making up your mind about it. Follow your own lead and don't limit your shopping to only those scents your friends use.

6. Experiment with fragrances. Even when you aren't really in the market for a new one, sample a couple of the new perfumes every now and again. Once you settle on a particular scent, you may find that you are drawn to other fragrances in the same family group. Women who favor gardenia, for example, often appreciate rose, lily-of-the-valley, and other floral scents as well. Remember, trying out new styles is the way to keep your fashion ideas up-to-date and the only way to build a flattering wardrobe. You should build your perfume wardrobe in the same manner. Then you can express your personality with fragrances just as you do with clothing.

FRAGRANCE LAYERING

Once you have chosen a scent, let yourself go —luxuriate in all of its many forms. Wear them all! This way of wearing fragrance is known in the beauty business as layering fragrance. For the fullest fragrance impression and the greatest enjoyment, use cologne and perfume together. Splash or spray cologne on body, neck, arms, and legs after bathing. Follow with perfume stroked on at the pulse points: temples, backs of the ears, base of the throat, over the collarbone, inside the elbows, backs of the wrists, backs of the knees, and backs of the ankles.

Layering, like so many other beautiful things, might begin in the bath. Use perfumed soap and a matching perfumed bath oil. Follow the bath with a matching fragrance in body lotion and talc, then cologne and perfume. And freshen fragrance periodically (as often as you re-apply lipstick is a handy rule of thumb) from a purse spray or other portable form.

Use your favorite scent in all its forms to create a subtle, delicious shimmer of fragrance that wraps you invisibly for hours.

ENJOY FRAGRANCE ALL AROUND YOU

You can extend the pleasures of fragrance to every corner of your life. It can be an enjoyable challenge to your creativity to make the whole house smell wonderful, filled with small surprises of scent.

Flowers and flowering plants are a natural. But there is an artistry involved in decorating with highly scented flowers. The perfume of flowers makes a perfect welcome to guests, and a bouquet or a flowering potted plant in the entrance hall is always a good idea. Just as a hallway is a good place to use brilliant colors that may be too bright for a room in which you spend long periods of time, so too the flowers with intense and haunting perfumes are good choices for an entryway. A tiny bouquet of white freesia, or stephanotis, or perhaps a potted hyacinth in early spring, will perfume a large area, yet they might overwhelm the sense of smell if used in the living room or the bedroom. Flowers make a beautiful centerpiece for the dining room table, but choose those that don't have a heavy fragrance, like camellias and chrysanthemums. Their perfume interferes with the aromas of food and drink. Or use fruits instead.

For those who live in northern cities, flowers may be a costly luxury for most of the year. Consider other forms of fragrant decoration: the attractive artificial pomander can be an amusing long-term addition to the looks and aroma of a room. Several pineapples in a low bowl symbolize hospitality and will perfume a room with island fragrance. Ripe apples or pears can be the source of a wonderfully comforting fragrance.

Artificial flowers might be your solution to colorful decoration. One well-known hostess kept enormous bouquets of silk flowers in her home, yet the scent of roses came from these arrangements of artificial blooms. The secret was a regular spraying with a discreet amount of rose perfume.

Don't forget bowls of potpourri here and there throughout the house. It's a pretty, old-fashioned, but effective, way of adding nice smells to your life. Explore the idea of making your own potpourri if you have a garden of fragrant roses for drying.

Below is a list of some other tricks with environmental aromas.

10 TIPS FOR SURROUNDING YOURSELF WITH FRAGRANT DELIGHTS

1. Tuck sachets in among the sheets and towels in the linen closet.
2. Before touching up washable clothes, spray a little cologne on the ironing board; but don't spray fragrance directly on clothes—it may spot.
3. Add a few drops of bath oil to a pot of simmering water, turn off the flame, and let the pot stand. You will add humidity to the atmosphere, and that's good for your skin. You also make a fragrant air that refreshes the whole house.
4. Save empty perfume and cologne bottles and leave them, caps off, at the bottom of the clothes hamper.
5. Tuck unwrapped perfumed guest soaps in your luggage before storing it. Bags will smell delicious, not musty, next time you pack for a trip.
6. Hang sachets on the coat hangers in your closet. Just two or three will make a whole closetful of clothes smell nice.
7. Some beauty companies provide attractive scented paper as fragrance samples. Save these and tuck them in your lingerie drawer. Or make them by saturating white blotter paper with your favorite fragrance.
8. Use closet pomanders and room pomanders all over the house. Amplify their aroma with cotton balls sprinkled with a drop of bath oil and tucked away in corners of the closets. A cotton ball saturated with bath oil and put in a decorative vase or bowl will scent the air in a subtle way when placed in an inconspicuous location, such as the upper shelf of a bookcase.
9. For a quick refresher, don't forget room-freshener sprays. Keep them handy all over the house. And don't forget a room-freshener to tuck in the glove compartment of the car.
10. To be soothed with lovely smells as you travel put a pomander in your car.

Of course, these few tips are only a springboard for your imagination. Once you try a couple of them, you will probably find yourself coming up with half a dozen more on your own. Soon, you will become skillful at using just a faint whiff of fragrance to give a little lift to every area of your life. Wherever you go, you will leave behind you, like footprints in the sand, a gentle reminder of a very special you.

A last word on new beginnings

Now, you know a lot about beauty, about being vibrantly healthy. You have the facts and the techniques; but even more important, you now know more about yourself. Just by reading this book you have inevitably been learning about your looks and have begun to get acquainted with yourself in a fresh new way. Now is the time to begin to use all this new information to make your own exciting statement, to face the world with the look of the '80s —what we at Avon call "naturalness with style."

Naturalness with style is the flair and vitality of today's woman, a fashion look that is relaxed, current and fresh. It's the open way you communicate with people, your special enthusiasm for life—all the qualities that make you unique.

You are ready to step forth into the world, radiating that glow and self-confidence that comes from knowing you never looked so good. But this is only the beginning.

It is difficult to form new beauty habits so thoroughly that they become automatic. And it is easy to slip back into the old, unbeautiful ways. That is why continuous self-assessment is so important. It takes a little time but will make a big difference. You must promise yourself to:

1. *Keep a weekly date with yourself for your Beauty Time. It will take you through the whole week in a well-groomed confident way.*

2. *Keep your new beauty notebook with you at all times and use it. The more often you refer to your record of your goals and habits, the clearer you will see the real you—and the easier it will be to make the outer you a more perfect expression of your ideal self.*

3. *Keep going. Don't give up or mininize your dreams, no matter how unattainable they might seem at the start. Your first attempt at a new way of doing eye makeup might be a disappointment. But if so, wash that false start away and begin again. You learn a little with every fresh try. Next time, or the next, you'll get it right and the flattering result will make all the determination seem worthwhile. Remember, becoming more attractive is an evolving and ongoing process. The wonderful part is that you can make progress every day by going forward in a gradual and natural way. Experiment and you will keep discovering new ways to improve your appearance. You'll not only look good, but feel beautiful . . . every day of your life.*

LOOKING GOOD, FEELING BEAUTIFUL

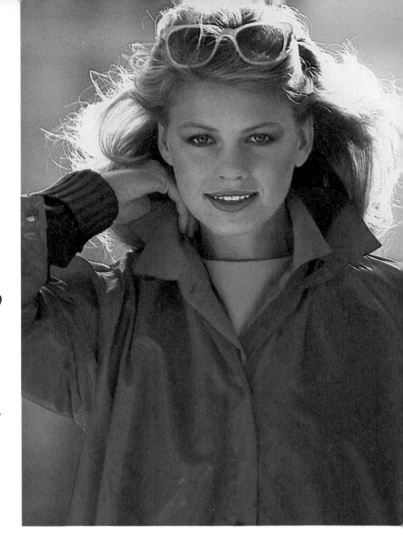

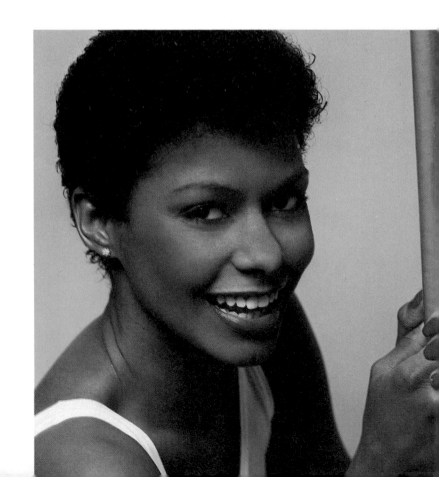